THE
GREAT
AGE
REB🌀🌀T

THE
GREAT
AGE
REB⚙️⚙️T

Cracking the Longevity Code
for a Younger Tomorrow

MICHAEL F. ROIZEN, M.D.
Peter Linneman, Ph.D.
Albert Ratner

With Ted Spiker

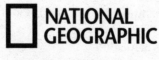
NATIONAL
GEOGRAPHIC

Washington, D.C.

Since 1888, the National Geographic Society has funded more than 14,000 research, conservation, education, and storytelling projects around the world. National Geographic Partners distributes a portion of the funds it receives from your purchase to National Geographic Society to support programs including the conservation of animals and their habitats.

Get closer to National Geographic Explorers and photographers, and connect with our global community. Join us today at nationalgeographic.com/join

For rights or permissions inquiries, please contact National Geographic Books Subsidiary Rights: bookrights@natgeo.com

Library of Congress Cataloging-in-Publication Data
Names: Roizen, Michael F., author. | Linneman, Peter, author. | Ratner, Albert, author. | Spiker, Ted, author.
Title: The great age reboot : cracking the longevity code for a younger tomorrow / Michael F. Roizen, M.D., Peter Linneman, Ph.D., Albert Ratner with Ted Spiker.
Description: Washington, DC : National Geographic, [2022] | Includes bibliographical references and index. | Summary: "As the human lifespan expands and more people are living to 100 years and beyond, New York Times best-selling author Michael Roizen, M.D., explains how to prepare for a longer, healthier future"-- Provided by publisher.
Identifiers: LCCN 2021031353 (print) | LCCN 2021031354 (ebook) | ISBN 9781426221514 (hardcover) | ISBN 9781426221521 (ebook)
Subjects: LCSH: Longevity. | Aging--Prevention. | Self-care, Health.
Classification: LCC RA776.75 .R647 2022 (print) | LCC RA776.75 (ebook) | DDC 612.6/8--dc23
LC record available at https://lccn.loc.gov/2021031353
LC ebook record available at https://lccn.loc.gov/2021031354

Printed in the United States of America

22/WOR/1

CONTENTS

Bodybuilding Supplement Promotes Healthy Aging and Extends Life Span, at Least in Mice
—Science

New Molecule Reverses Alzheimer's-Like Memory Decline
—Neuroscience News

A Cure for Heart Disease? A Single Shot Succeeds in Monkeys
—New York Times

Neuron Breakthrough Raises Hope for Possible Parkinson's Treatment
—Financial Times

A Research Team Builds Robots From Living Cells
—The Economist

A Missing Gene Could Restore His Sight
—Bloomberg

Israeli Scientists Claim to Reverse Aging Process
—Jerusalem Post

Lab-Grown Heart Cells Implanted Into Human Patient for the First Time
—New Atlas

Biologists Identify Pathways That Extend Life Span by 500 Percent
—Phys.org

I'm Testing an Experimental Drug to See If It Halts Alzheimer's
—New Scientist

We May Not Have to Age So Fast
—Wall Street Journal

Drug Reverses Age-Related Cognitive Decline Within Days
—Medical Xpress

Yale scientists repair injured spinal cords using patients' own stem cells
—Journal of Clinical Neurology and Neurosurgery

PREFACE

LATE IN 2020, HEADLINES SWIRLED AROUND THE HEALTH story of the year—probably the health story of the decade. The world was focused on vaccines and ventilators, on death rates and masking guidelines. COVID-19 consumed us—and for good reason.

But for the better part of that year and the previous two (and really, since I had graduated from medical school), I had spent much of my time looking at the other end of the spectrum—the jaw-dropping medical, technological, and scientific advances that were about to significantly extend lives, rather than shorten them.

Over the course of my career, I had immersed myself in stem cells, genetics, robots, and more. But I wanted to see some of these new game-changers in action. So, one day in December 2020, I walked about a half-mile on the Cleveland Clinic Skyway from my office to the 3D Print Lab of the Lerner Research Institute at the clinic. There, I met with Ryan Klatte, its principal research engineer and director. He holds a Ph.D. in engineering and loves talking about the 3D printing of organs.

Around the lab—about the size of a modest living room— Ryan showed me the group's printers, as well as a few of the model organs and body parts they had produced. Pediatric hearts with complex congenital abnormalities, a pancreas with a specific tumor close to a bile duct, a kidney with arterial abnormalities, fatty tissue for a breast reconstruction, an aneurysm. They had all been modeled from CT and MRI scans of real people, with the tissues in question printed with different color resins. This way, a surgeon could examine the model in three dimensions and make decisions based on the patient's specific anatomy—before operating.

Ryan showed me a model of a liver from a potential donor. The colored resins clearly showed where veins, bile ducts, and vessels resided, so that surgeons would know exactly where to cut to avoid hitting parts of the circulatory or biliary systems that could cause life-threatening damage.

Though all human anatomy is essentially the same, there are some minor differences—placement of fat, the road map of blood and bile vessels—from person to person. When doctors can see the organ (or tumor or tissue) in three dimensions before they operate, they are able to design an efficient, effective, and safe surgical strategy (especially in cases with challenging or distorted anatomy). These 3D models were saving people's lives in ways that were never possible before.

But that's not where the story ends. It's actually where it begins.

What if that same 3D printer could produce not only models of organs, but the organs themselves? Now, plastic thrown into recycling bins is transformed into resin to build replicas. But what if unwanted fat from liposuction operations could be "reprinted" as a new heart or breast? What if these printers could use young cells to print actual organs, cells, and tissues—any you need—to replace the dysfunctional ones?

This process, of course, would be incredibly complex. But in essence, here's what it would involve:

1. Filling the printer's cartridges with three or more kinds of cells: those of the tissue or organ being created, and those forming vessels and nerves needed to connect it to the body.
2. Printing a matrix in the shape of the organ, made of biodegradable material, that would stand in for that organ until the cells could grow into it and take over.

This could be our future.

Development of this kind of technology is now happening all over the world. And so is work on many other major advances that are about to fundamentally change the way we approach medicine and health.

That's what this book is about—the "what ifs" that are knocking on society's door.

What if . . . we could replace organs by printing new ones?

What if . . . we could reprogram our dying cells to be youthful ones?

What if . . . we could rewrite our DNA to lead us to a healthier future?

Not only would we live longer, but we would live younger. In 1998, we believed age 60 could be the new 40. In 2030, that potential expands dramatically: 90 could be the new 40. Old age wouldn't be, well, old.

Of the 14 major areas of new research developing around longevity (see pages 59–60), there will be a few treatments that become commonplace and help you stay younger longer (while it's impossible to predict which ones, we have our guesses). Those advances will exponentially change society and our economy and will also change you and your future.

My co-authors, Peter Linneman, Ph.D., and Albert Ratner, and I refer to this transformation as the Great Age Reboot. This book contains our research explaining what that reboot means for you: what breakthroughs are on the horizon, and what you can do to prepare for the coming shift.

Longer lives made possible with these medical breakthroughs will be healthier and more productive lives, which will have a major benefit to the economy. As a result of large population increases due to greater longevity, and the increase in productive human capital, the economy will present much greater opportunities for humanity, and for solving inequalities. (Yes, government policies are going to have to keep up—when 90 is the new 40, the Congressional Budget Office will have to stop thinking that everyone over 65 is only a cost to society.) The Great Age Reboot is coming—and it's coming fast. Now is the time to prepare for the crucial decisions that will come with it, and for the youth and joy that will be yours to achieve if you want them.

We look forward to joining you on this unprecedented journey.

—Michael F. Roizen, M.D.
Chief Wellness Officer Emeritus, Cleveland Clinic

WHAT IS THE GREAT AGE REBOOT ALL ABOUT?

SOMETIME IN THE NOT-TOO-DISTANT FUTURE, our medical landscape will look like this:

- You will 3D-print a new organ to replace a diseased one.[1]
- A robot will remove plaque from your arteries, and you will not need stent surgery.[2]
- If you have the gene that shows you're predisposed to colon cancer, a snip here, a snip there, and—*boom*—you will cut that gene out of your DNA. And colon cancer out of your future.[3] [4]

Some 100 years ago, most people couldn't imagine a world with antibiotics or immunizations, let alone MRI-guided robotic surgery performed on a patient in an operating room in Cleveland, Tennessee, by a surgeon in Cleveland, Ohio. But these breakthroughs are all very real—and are becoming commonplace—in modern medicine.

So today, while you might not be able to fathom the robotic surgery, gene editing, and other incredible medical advances that await us, they are coming.

In fact, in some cases, they're already here.[5]

That's because we are now living on the cusp of the Great Age Reboot: a period of scientific and intellectual advancements that will not only change the way we live, feel, and act, but transform our culture as we know it. Believe it or not, within the next 10 years the world will rocket into new norms of aging, new population increases, new life spans, and new ways of living. The changes will be radical, and they will come fast.

In developed countries today, the average life expectancy at birth is about 81; a few people live until about 110, and, in extreme cases, 120-plus. But our projections, based on scientific advances in the major areas of aging research, show that by 2030 you will be able to slow your rate of aging—likely to an average life expectancy for those now over 40 to at least 108.

And down the line, it will not be uncommon for people to regularly live to 115 and even 130. That jump—from 81 to 108, 27 or more years of living in just 10 years—is unprecedented, representing a 1,100 percent increase over the two-and-a-half-year average gain we've obtained per decade for the last 140 years.

You may be asking, what does this look like? After all, who wants to live longer if it just means living older?

Nobody.

But hear us out: This aging boom will actually lead to more "prime-living" years, not "elderly," downtrodden ones. Think of it this way: You won't just be living longer. Instead, you'll be extending the period between ages 30 and 60 to between 30 and 90.

And here's another way to think about it: Your 20s will last maybe 15 or 20 years. Same goes for your 30s and 40s. In fact, there's a very high chance that sometime between 2025 and 2035, the typical 95-year-old will look and function more like the typical 50-year-old of today.

What this means in practice is that a person's biological age, or "RealAge,"* could be half that of her calendar, or actual, age—assuming that person has made advantageous health and lifestyle choices.[6]

And wait, there's more: In the not-so-distant future, 95 won't be an upper age range; it will have become the norm. Of course, if you're older today, the window of your aging potential is smaller. But happily, all of us have the ability to make changes that can lead to a longer and healthier life. That's because the key to these mind-boggling numbers is not your calendar age, but how you live and feel.

So when it comes to the Great Age Reboot, the question isn't whether you want to live to 110 or longer. Rather, it's whether you want your 20s through your 70s to be extended so that you have more years feeling better and younger. In Japan, as well as in many other countries and cultures, people have embraced this concept of "young old," or "yold," meaning old in years but young in feeling, looks, and function.[7]

In short, we believe that longevity is not only the next disruptor, but the greatest disruptor ever. It has the potential to cause changes even more sweeping and powerful than the invention of the chip (micro, not potato!) 60 years ago.[8]

---

* RealAge was developed by Mike Roizen—using thousands of scientific studies—to show how your body could act if it were an age different from your calendar age (younger or older), based on dozens of your lifestyle choices and biomarkers.

The Great Age Reboot will be defined by advances that will extend your life and improve its quality in what will seem like incredible ways.

Ultimately, though, living longer—and being both healthier and wealthier while you do so—has a lot to do with you. *You* must make good choices now. *You* must take care of your body and brain. *You* must save wisely every day. The healthier you are when these revolutionary changes arrive, the more they can help you.

Therefore, we believe that in order to benefit fully, you have to prepare yourself for the coming reboot. And that's what this book will do: reveal what's on the horizon, explain how it will enrich your life, and unveil what you can do today to be ready for the future and make sure you get the fun and joy of it.[9] [10]

To help you prepare for the Great Age Reboot, we're going to break this book into four sections:

In **Part 1**, we'll explore the origins of longevity and give some of our predictions for the future.

In **Part 2**, we'll look at some of the most fascinating and promising medical breakthroughs.

In **Part 3**, we'll take a step back so we can see the big picture: what these important changes mean for our bodies, our economy, and our society as a whole.

And finally, in **Part 4**, we'll offer a customized plan to help *you* prepare for, embrace, and enjoy the Great Age Reboot.

Let's face it: Big changes are afoot. We are in the midst of an extraordinary biological and societal revolution that is affecting human life span even as we write. Sure, it may be difficult to picture a youthful 95-year-old. But you know what? In the 1930s, few could picture a youthful 65. Someone in the early 1900s never could have imagined living until 80.[11]

Will you decide to change with the times? Will you prepare to stay younger longer by extending the good years? And will you help society change?

As we stand on the brink of the Great Age Reboot, those decisions are yours to make.

PART 1

YESTERDAY TO TOMORROW

How the history of medical breakthroughs reveals something about our future

We are all living longer. Since the 1800s people in developed countries have gained a few years of life expectancy every decade.[1] But with revolutionary breakthroughs in science now available and many more in the pipeline, we are seeing fun-filled, healthy life extension of 20 to 30 years or more—perhaps as soon as the 2030s. Within that window, it will be commonplace for people to live to 120 and beyond.

The COVID-19 pandemic that killed so many people around the globe in 2020 and beyond will not change the overall growth of longevity rates. According to data from Johns Hopkins University at the time we were writing this book, the United States had already far surpassed the cumulative number of coronavirus deaths (more than one million) that would lower the life expectancy at birth for 2021 by one full year, lower than any year since 2003.[2] In fact, in early 2021, the federal government reported that the pandemic had indeed steeply reduced average life spans for Americans by a full year over the course of less than 12 months, from 78.8 years in 2019 to 77.3 years in 2020.[3]

By comparison, the country's infamous opioid crisis led to an average 0.4-year (153 days) decline in life expectancy at birth annually. And at its peak, the HIV epidemic reduced the U.S. life expectancy at birth by 0.3 year in a single year, from 1992 to 1993.

Of course, any longevity drop feels concerning. But as it happens, unless deaths reach four million or greater in the United States (or 80 million worldwide) U.S. life expectancy at birth is expected to revert to 2010 levels by the end of 2025, assuming the world receives vaccines effective for all of the SARS-CoV-2 variants by 2023. If this comes to pass, the U.S. life expectancy at birth will continue its upward trajectory. Global pandemics are certainly daunting, and this one has already demonstrated how important it is to take care of yourself.

That means that despite what we have experienced with COVID-19, there is vast potential for extending lives in unprecedented ways—whether we're talking about the 3D printing of organs or creating a bionic human.

Why are these scenarios so difficult to envision? Because human beings tend to think in linear terms: If you have to walk a mile and you take 30 linear steps, you're, well, approximately 30 yards (or meters) closer to completing that mile. By the same token, it's difficult to see that a society in the midst of a generational medical crisis—both the tragedies of the pandemic and also the ongoing crises of widespread obesity, diabetes, arthritis, dementia, and more—is in fact close to wiping out today's most dangerous killers.

But technology and science don't always work linearly. They can work *exponentially*. That is, one advance doesn't lead to two, then three. One step leads to two, then four, then eight, and so on. It's like taking leaps, rather than steps—exponential leaps. Where 30 literal steps may get you 100 or so feet (30 yards or meters), 30 exponential steps would take you 26 times around the world.[3] And that's how the science of aging has and will continue to advance.

We are on the verge of *exponential* changes in both medical advancements and increased life spans. Science is changing the ways we are able to manipulate our cells and our DNA. But not to fix a problem (as in the case of antibiotics) or to detect a problem before it gets bad (as in the case of MRIs). Instead, these changes will change *us* by changing how we operate at a core level.

Before we get to the rapid advances, let's take a look at where we've been—and where we're headed.

CHAPTER 1

LOOKING BACK TO LOOK FORWARD

The longevity landscape of 1900 to 2020 has set us up for the future

Every day, we're inundated with various forms of history. Maybe your bookshelf includes a biography of Ben Franklin. Maybe you hunker down with the National Geographic Channel (which often has more history than the History Channel) or are addicted to PBS or Netflix documentaries. Or maybe history is just a part of your everyday life, and you don't even give it much thought: a family history at the doctor's office, an order history on your Starbucks app. History matters because it informs our present, predicts our future, inspires change, and gives us context about the world around us.

This observation also applies to longevity. Yes, this book is about looking ahead to your future—what you need to do to extend your young years, your most productive years, for as long as you can and with as much fun, energy, passion, and joy as possible. But to understand the future and what it all means, you must first look back—not only at the timeline of longevity, but also at the medical advances that have coincided with our increasing life spans. There's a reason we have rearview mirrors: Important stuff happens behind us, even as we're driving forward. Grasping what the future holds requires an appreciation of the past.

In this chapter, we'll consider longevity through the lens of personal and medical history to help you understand the larger context of how and why scientific advances have made it possible. Finally, we'll use the past to set up the future, explaining the current lines of scientific thinking relevant to longevity and what that means going forward.

Make no mistake: It's not easy to predict the future. The truth is, we can never truly know what awaits (can you imagine how 1930s Depression-era citizens might have processed drone deliveries?). But we can still have a strong sense about where we're going by looking at where we've been.

The tricky part of this whole conversation is that age is a moving target. If you're reading this book at the age of 20, you will be contemplating an entirely different scenario than someone who is reading it at age 50 or 80. But the good news is that we'll be giving you smart information about the Great Age Reboot no matter how old you are. Down the line you will likely be able to reboot your life and body to return it to its younger, more optimal years, eliminate most of your past mistakes, and start again as if you're much younger, all with the knowledge of your history and that of past generations.

But here's what to remember now: Just as the average life span is different today than it was on the day you were born, average life span will increase as you get older. This chart will help you visualize what your future could look like with the new scientific advances that are coming:

GAR FOR LIFE EXPECTANCY
IN THE UNITED STATES

Your Approximate Age in 2022	Average Life Span Predicted for You When You Were Born (female)*	Predicted Average Life Span for You in 2030 (GARP—Great Age Reboot Predictions)	Additional Years for You to Live as of 2022
25	79	125	100
35	78	122	87
45	77	120	75
55	74	115	60
65	73	110	45
75	68	100	25

* In general, for males, subtract three years from all figures.[1]

To help this feel more concrete, take the examples of this book's three co-authors. Albert was born in 1927, with a life expectancy at birth of just 57.[2] If that had come to pass, he would have missed George Bush 1 and 2, Clinton, Obama, and both the Trump and the Biden years, stents, statins, immuno-therapy, and COVID-19 (not to mention the iPad, the iPhone, Siri, and Alexa, which he uses daily). He's already lived to age 94, more than 64 percent longer than he was expected to at birth. Meanwhile, Mike's life expectancy at birth in 1946 was 71—an age he's already passed. He looks forward to his reboot, as does Peter, who is 71.

This change in longevity and how this disruptor will affect us won't wait till 2050—it is happening now and will affect population dynamics in the United States, as shown in this chart, very soon (even now):

LONGEVITY IS THE NEXT DISRUPTOR™ IN NUMBERS TO 2050*

Age	2020 Great Age Reboot Population (millions)	2030 Great Age Reboot Population (millions)	2040 Great Age Reboot Population (millions)	2050 Great Age Reboot Population (millions)	2050 U.S. Census Bureau Population (millions)
0–9	40.7	41.5	42.4	**43.3**	43.3
10–19	42.4	42.8	43.2	**43.9**	43.9
20–29	45.4	46.1	46.8	**47.3**	47.3
30–39	44.7	47.2	48.6	**49.7**	48.7
40–49	40.7	43.9	47.2	**50.5**	49.0
50–59	42.7	45.0	47.4	**50.8**	48.4
60–69	39.4	41.7	43.9	**46.1**	43.1
70–79	25.0	29.5	37.2	**37.6**	33.3
80–89	10.3	18.8	29.3	**35.0**	23.6
90–99	2.3	7.8	15.0	**29.1**	7.9
100–109	0	1.8	6.2	**13.0**	0.4
110–119	0	0	0.9	**4.1**	0
120+	0	0	0	**0.5**	0
Totals	**333.6**	**366.1**	**408.1**	**451.0**	**388.9**
Population increase over prior decades (Total 117.5 to 2050)					
		32.5	**42.0**	**42.9**	
Cumulative Great Age Reboot population increase from 2020 32%					
		32.5	**74.6**	**117.5**	

* All U.S. Census data used in this book are based on 2019 data and projections.

We project higher population rates not because of increased births, but because of a lower death rate brought upon by medical advances. So our projection of a U.S.

population of 451 million in 2050? We estimate 316.5 million of those people are already alive. That is, 70 percent of the 2050 population is already living. As a point of reference, the U.S. population is 333 million. We predict 85 percent of this population will still be alive in 2050. Stated differently, the growth of the population by 2050 will reflect far more on the change in the death rate than on births. Let's unpack this a bit.

In 2019, U.S. Census actuaries project that in 2050, the U.S. population will be about 55.3 million higher than it is today, reaching a level of about 390 million. Others think it will be less due to changes in fertility. They in fact argue that life expectancy is declining in developed countries.

In addition to the COVID-19 pandemic, we've been living in the United States with the epidemics of opioid abuse, depression with an increase in suicides, and obesity and its medical consequences. But over the course of the year before COVID-19 hit, medical science, public health, and personal behaviors had changed enough for life expectancy to increase again. This trend reveals that you can, in fact, influence some aspects of your own life expectancy through your personal choices.

While life-expectancy decreases have happened in every prior pandemic studied (and we now have an epidemic and a pandemic in the United States—opioid addiction and SARS-CoV-2), life expectancy has rebounded fast in the past: In 1917 average life expectancy at birth was 48 for men and 54 for women, which declined by 12 years to 36 for men and 42 for women by the end of 1918 (the year the Spanish flu pandemic hit) but rebounded to 54 for men and 56 for women by 1920.[34]

We believe that immigration will also rebound over time (as it does in waves), and fertility rates will stabilize at lower levels. And when we adjust these estimates to reflect longer, rebooted life expectancies, we think this growth will not be 55 million as predicted by U.S. Census actuaries (who have been wrong in the past) or 36 million in the recent projection in *The Lancet*.[5] We believe that it will be closer to 117.5 million, with the U.S. population likely to reach 451 million people.

For ease of understanding going forward, we will refer to our projections as GARP, or Great Age Reboot Projections. We are not alone in questioning the very conservative projections of those actuaries; the Pew Research Center has made projections closer to ours, at over 438 million, an increase of 105 million, attributing much of the increase to immigration.[6] And while we do not know precisely what jobs will be available, we think there will be plenty, as every disruptor so far has created more opportunities (remember, when horses were replaced by autos, it was feared a lack of jobs would follow because fewer people would be needed to care for the horses or deal with their excrement in the streets; the opposite, of course, happened).

If you think we're crazy, just think about the chart on page 27—your expected life span at birth compared with what awaits now. And consider your longevity potential compared with that of families over the past century in the United States:

The Typical 1900 Family

The 40-year-old patriarch in all likelihood can trace his family tree back to the 1700s. His first wife died in childbirth, and he had one child die of rheumatic fever when she was a toddler. He works seven days a week to make the equivalent of about $10,000 (in today's dollars) annually. All of his kids—ranging from seven to 22—also have jobs so the family can support itself. The patriarch dies at age 45 after getting an infection that cannot be treated. He did not know any of his grandparents as an adult.

Average life span: 47 for white males, 49 for white females, 33 for black males, 34 for black females.

The Typical 1925 Family

This family is working and happy that all of the children can read and write. But they are familiar with loss because those kids have an uncle who was killed in World War I and an aunt who died in the Great Influenza epidemic (which killed about one percent of the U.S. population, equivalent to 3.3 million people today). The family is worried about their kids because this month, measles, mumps, chicken pox, and scarlet fever have ravaged their neighborhood. Sudden deaths from many causes are common.

Average life span: 57 for white males, 65 for white females, 46 for black males, 47 for black females.

The Typical 1950 Family

The mother worked during World War II at a bomb-making factory and has problems with memory due to an unexplained problem (now understood to be lead toxicity from the fumes involved with bomb and bullet manufacturing). The father worked on the Manhattan Project and later was diagnosed with thyroid cancer at age 60 as a result of the radiation involved in making the first atomic weapon. Sudden deaths, from such things as heart attacks, are still common. But life expectancy is longer due to public health measures, new medicines, new procedures, and vaccines that are being developed (it took 10 to 20 years to develop and test vaccines in this era). Surgery is becoming much safer as newer anesthesia techniques and surgical standards are being developed.

Average life span: 67 for white males, 72 for white females, 59 for black males, 63 for black females (that is, an additional 20 to 30 years over 50 years since 1900).

The Typical 1975 Family

The mother is one of the first women admitted to a previously all-male medical school and later in life, at age 67, she will work part-time for a large health system. At age 67, she is 20 pounds heavier than she was at her high school graduation and suffers from severe arthritis in her hips and knees; she is scheduled for a hip replacement in three months. Her husband worked as an engineer for United Technologies and then for four other companies as his company was sold three times. He retired two years ago with a small pension and Social Security. He is 40 pounds heavier than he was at his high school graduation, has type 2 diabetes, and received three bypasses for coronary artery disease. He takes care of his 93-year-old mother, who lives on the first floor of their home and is losing her memory and cognitive abilities. They will have three children who in 2022 are in their 40s.

Average life span: 69.5 for white males, 77 for white females, 62 for black males, 71 for black females.

The Typical 2000 Family

Both parents are in their second marriages, with blended families. Blended families have expanded family trees, but generally, large families are uncommon, as fertility rates have declined steadily since the early 1970s. The mother has gone through four operations to repair knee cartilage, and the dad takes medication for heart disease. Sudden deaths are rare in this era, but the aging parents are seeing the detrimental health effects of a society with more and more processed foods and climbing obesity rates.

Average life span: 75 for white males, 80 for white females, 68 for black males, 75 for black females (a rise of 8 to 12 years over 50 years).

The Typical 2020 Family

Both parents are working. Mom works in HR at a robotics manufacturing plant; Dad works as a security officer for Facebook, weeding out terrorist posts and sites. They met at an online-security job-listing symposium in 2017. They have two generations of children—one from their first marriages and another set of children 15 years later from this, their second marriage. Most children have living grandparents, and many have living great-grandparents. Fertility rates have continued to decline, taking a major drop during the recession of 2008–2009 and not recovering as well as after past economic downturns. Sudden deaths are common only from gun violence and severe drug abuse. Rates for obesity (now a condition for over 43 percent of all over age 19) are soaring, as is predisposition to heart disease and type 2 diabetes, but medication is helping assuage the effects.

Average life span: 76 for white males, 81 for white females, 72 for black males, 79 for black females (both men's groups pulled down by the opioid deaths of young males).

So, over the past 120 years, life expectancy in the U.S. has increased by over 36 years, first because of better sanitation and other public health measures, and then because of better treatment of childhood diseases. More recently, life expectancy has increased due to treatment and management of chronic diseases that usually develop in adults.[3] And human well-being and living standards, as exemplified by these family stories, have continually improved to levels unimaginable in the 30 years prior. We expect that improvement to continue and accelerate because we as a culture are—for the first time ever—focusing on the medical problems of the aged and the basic mechanisms of aging. Until now, we have focused efforts on the young and prime-aged, as is evident from the Longevity Timeline that follows.

The Longevity Timeline: Major Medical Advances

Around 1920, the world's view of longevity shifted forever. Until then, the prevailing view was that humans were made with only so much juice in them; we had a limited capacity for life—only so many beats of your heart—and would die when the time came, when we had used up those beats. But the realization in the 1920s that life could be extended through scientific advances was a game-changer. Now sanitation and medicine weren't just about delaying death; they were about extending and improving life. That shift in attitude set up what is happening today: advances that will ultimately lead to exponential increases in life span.

Instead of treating our bodies like they were built with a set number of years in them, we realized that we could act like medical puppeteers: We could save lives, we could extend lives, we could *fight* the inevitable by extending both the length and the quality of even the last few years. We could avoid chronic diseases and even reverse them and live "younger" every year.

The history of longevity is fascinating, documenting how increased life spans coincided with such advances as vaccines, antibiotics, and more. So, come with us for a quick ride down longevity lane, to see how far we've come—and be inspired by how far we'll be going.

THE LONGEVITY TIMELINE
MAJOR MEDICAL ADVANCES

1799	Average life span: 36. The first smallpox vaccine is introduced. This is the first major development in preventative health that extended life span.
1800s	Aspirin is born, based on Hippocrates' use of willow bark in ancient Greece. The implications decades later extend far beyond pain, to reducing the effects of some infections and preventing strokes, heart disease, dementia, and at least 13 types of cancer.
1846	The emergence of anesthetics makes surgical procedures more bearable and allows more intricate and successful procedures. Surgery no longer requires four strong men holding you down at home for a procedure that could last only 10 minutes at most.
1850	The five leading causes of death are infectious diseases: tuberculosis, dysentery, cholera, malaria, and typhoid fever.
1860s	Sanitation comes into the public health spotlight—and likely saves millions of lives, as many early deaths were attributed to unclean water and surroundings. Clean water allows effective hand washing, which becomes common thereafter, reducing transmission of infections.
1890s	Heart surgery is invented.

1900	Average life span: 47. Society lacks hospitals and medical facilities. Anesthesia and surgery are still risky and difficult. The five leading causes of death (pneumonia, tuberculosis, diarrhea, heart disease, and stroke) include three infectious diseases.
1907	The first antibiotic is created, marking the beginning of the discovery of the antibacterial power of drugs like penicillin to contribute to extending life expectancy and longevity.
1917–19	Spanish flu whips around Earth six times and kills one percent of the population, reducing life expectancy by eight to 12 years to under age 40. It recovers in three years, with life expectancy of 55 for Caucasian women at birth by 1923.
1920s	Vaccines are found to protect against such things as tuberculosis and pertussis.
1921	Insulin is discovered.
1928	Average life span: 55
1933	Not enough food for laboratory animals during the Great Depression leads to the discovery that calorie restriction in mice extends life span by over 30 percent.
1938	The federal Food, Drug, and Cosmetic Act is passed, making medication in the United States much more likely to benefit than harm users and their longevity.
1940s	Penicillin is introduced to treat infections.
1942	A prototype of the pacemaker is developed.
1947	The artificial kidney machine is invented. Enrollment for a study of the health behaviors and outcomes of members of Chicago public employee unions (gas, electric, and water companies) is in full swing. This study followed employees until death and demonstrated increased longevity (30 percent) and dramatically decreased medical costs (by 50 percent over the rest of their lives) for those employees with biomarkers and behaviors that fostered health long before retirement.

1954	The first successful organ transplant (a kidney) takes place.
1955	The first polio vaccine is available.
1960s	Vaccines for mumps and measles are introduced.
1967	CT scans allow views inside the body without surgery.
1975	Average life span: 72.6
1983	The Health Professionals and Nurses Health Studies are launched: These will begin to confirm that personal choices such as diet and amount of physical activity substantially (by 10 years each) influence longevity.
1990s	It's discovered that calorie restriction helps extend life in most species studied.
Mid-1990s	Statins are shown to decrease atherosclerosis.
2000	Average life span: 78
2000	The five leading causes of death are heart disease, cancer, stroke, lung disease, and accidents.
2002	Sugar is identified as a major cause of inflammatory diseases.
2003	The Human Genome Project is declared complete, paving the way for genetic advances that will have a profound impact on disease risk and longevity.
2006–2009	Cigarette laws and taxes are recognized as being effective at reducing smoking, a major cause of cancer.
2016	Taxation of sugary drinks, which can increase health risks, begins in major cities such as Berkeley, New York, and Philadelphia.
2016	Average life span: 80
2020	COVID-19 starts to increase the death rate of those over 70 and those with comorbidities of obesity, diabetes, hypertension, lung disease, and heart disease.

2020	Vaccine platforms are built in a matter of months for faster response to future viral invasions and hold the promise of reducing the effect of future pandemics on death rates. There are exponential gains in longevity in animals (by the equivalent of 30 to 70 human years) using stem cells, senolytics, and other advances in the major research areas of aging. We believe some of these approaches will make it through human safety and effectiveness testing to extend life expectancy by at least 30 years in a decade.
2021	COVID-19 drives U.S. life expectancy numbers down by more than a year, from 78.8 to 77.3, but the decrease is expected to be temporary as the population slowly gets vaccinated.

Redefining "Old"

Our belief: The lives of humans will be more unimaginable in 30 years than in any prior 30-year period. What Moore's Law states for computational productivity in the past 50 years (that is, that microchip speed increases while cost decreases) is about to occur for human-capital productivity (a measure of the economic value generated by the skills, education, capacity, and attributes of labor) in the next 30 years. Productive work life has increased 25 years in the last 100 years; we expect it to increase at least another 25 years in the next 10 to 30 years.

Given this, perhaps the most important point to make is that you must be open to new paradigms. On the face of it, the prospect of living to 130 or beyond may not sound all that appealing—especially if it means that your dinner consists of puréed peas, that you can't hear the night nurse tell you that they're puréed peas and not pistachio pudding, and that you can't remember if you even like peas—or, for that matter, if you have children.

But that is not the future that longevity holds.

Think of this new world as your own personal version of the

Hippocratic oath, which implores health professionals to "do no harm." You are about to become your own personal professional to help your other professionals. During the Great Age Reboot, we should all be adhering to the same principle. Think of it as the Reboot oath: Do no harm through your daily lifestyle choices and decisions you make every day (this is the subject of Part 4). In the past, as life expectancy has increased, per capita income and well-being (and joy of living) for individuals and societies have increased and social inequality has decreased. So when expanding the window of your productive years (effectively, finding that fountain of your prime years) is the norm, you and the world will thrive physically and economically, and we'll have the real opportunity to decrease social inequality.

After looking at the timeline of advances, it may be tempting to sit back and wait for technology to come up with a magical device that will keep us healthy, no matter what we ingest or how little we exercise. But we also need to help ourselves—and that is the foundation of this book. Specifically, that means the following:

1. Personal decisions (good and bad) matter more when the consequences last longer. Imagine a time when the life expectancy was 50 (or even younger). Bad lifestyle decisions may have decreased your ultimate longevity—but they also didn't matter as much, since you didn't have to live with the consequences for long.

But what happens when you make bad lifestyle decisions and now, because of various medical advances, your life has been extended? That means you're in for more years with a lower quality of life.

Say you make a choice—say, with poor eating habits that lead to being overweight—that decreases your energy level. Now, instead of living with lower energy for, say, 10 years, you have to live with lower energy for 80 years. Or consider age-related weight gain. Most people gain an average of 1.25 pounds a year as they get older (that is the national average in the United States and the international average for all developed countries).[7] [8] [9] While that might not seem like much to contend with between the ages of 45 and 75, what if that creep happens between the ages of 45 and 120? That's a lot more weight—94 extra pounds versus 37—along with the additional medical and lifestyle burdens that come with it. And 30 extra pounds for the average 60-year-old increased their risk of hospitalization from COVID-19 more than twofold, from 3.6 to 7.2 percent, and greatly increased the likelihood of fatality.[10]

So now flip that scenario around: Make good choices, and you'll live that same extended life with more vibrancy, potency, energy, and joy. Your good decisions last longer—making a longer life a *younger* life. The choice is yours.

2. Hospitals will need to change. They were once considered places to die, and then as places to have a chance to heal from catastrophic wounds, and then as places to be treated with antibiotics for major infections and radical surgery for major injuries, and then as places where minimal medicines and minor surgeries can make major changes.

Societally, we will need to see shifts in how we—including the medical community—approach wellness. Instead of hospitals being repositories for the sick, they will need to become wellness centers after recovery or treatment reverses major issues. That is, they will need to focus on prevention, on health optimization, on opportunities to reboot our bodies. Many more people will recover from illness at home, as hospitals will bring those facilities and services to you, and less expensively. Note: With a decrease in fertility we expect more stabilization of pediatric and delivery centers, and with an increase in longevity we will see growth of plastic surgery and cosmetic procedures.

When hospitals and reconceived drugstores like CVS and Walgreens become more like wellness centers than treatment centers, we stop becoming a reactive culture when it comes to medicine and become more proactive—taking our health and wellness seriously before problems start.

This shift in thinking and in practice is a necessary part of the development of the reboot, as it will create a partnership between the individual and the medical community to fully and holistically think about health and longevity.

3. *This great societal disruptor will have bumps, but every day, on average, will be a positive for society.* Every social disruptor takes some getting used to (remember the first cell phones, TVs, and computers?). The same applies to the Great Age Reboot. This shift in life expectancy will affect the economy, health care systems, insurance, government policy, and family structure ("Yes, your great-great-great grandma is coming to your birthday party; she's driving Grandma"). Change is not easy. But it's important to remember that society will benefit from this larger shift, because it will ensure more and better human capital (a measure of the skills, education, capacity, and attributes of labor that influence people's productive capacity and earning)—and human capital pays for itself.

How? Let's follow the money:

- If each of today's 150 million workers in the U.S. worked one more day a year because of a healthier life, at about $600 in gross domestic product (GDP) per worker per day, those additional days would generate about $90 billion additional GDP annually—meaning $15 billion in federal tax revenue and almost $9 billion in taxes for state and local governments.

- And if each of the 24 million workers over the age of 55 who works today worked just one year longer due to improved health (say, until age 66 instead of 65), it would increase the GDP by $340 billion annually and federal government revenue by almost $60 billion.

- If those same workers held jobs for five more years, the impact approaches $1.5 trillion in GDP per year. And this is easily achievable due to the Great Age Reboot, particularly since greater health means fewer of today's workers will die prematurely. In fact, our predictions of a 2.5 percent growth rate are conservative.

- Another way of understanding this concept is that currently the typical worker has a typical work life of about 40 years. If they work just one more year, that is a 2.5 percent increase in their work life. If they work just four more years, it is a 10 percent increase in their work life. And since these additional work years will come later in their careers, they will be in their most productive work years due to the knowledge and judgment obtained over those years. This means that a 2.5 percent or 10 percent increase in their work lives will generate much greater increases in their lifetime output (and taxes paid).

These additional resources will more than pay for the extra costs of unilaterally increased life expectancy.[11] In every society in the past, longevity of the population improves individual and societal economics (longevity is a stronger influence even than education). And if we use these extra resources wisely, we can afford longer and healthier lives. (In fact, if we are going to live 25 to 30 more healthy years, it would make sense that we'd choose to work an extra five to 15 years.)

In this brave new world, human capital will become ours to create, maintain, and harvest. And this means that we not only can afford longevity; we cannot afford to turn our backs on longevity. Of course, government policies such as age-of-retirement payments will need to change. This new workforce—of older people who work as if their calendar age were much younger—will experience increased productivity and longer work lives, while enjoying more disability-free time, expending more consumer activity, and generating high tax proceeds. It's win-win for everyone.

Even if we are wrong and only the current linear longevity trends continue, it means that today's 20-year-olds will be able to live healthy lives into their early 90s. And if the emerging medical research associated with aging mechanisms plays out over the next 15 years, these 20-year-olds will live to 110, effectively gaining three more years in each decade of their lives. This will unleash massive economic growth as the workforce collectively experiences a longer "prime." And the rest of us will have the energy to consume more and longer, which in turn generates the need for new jobs and increased output.

This growth will easily pay for our longevity, just as it has done since the late 1800s, when human life span began increasing. Since 1880, the life expectancy of newborns has increased 2.5 years on average every decade. This new population has not been and will not be broken-down drains on society; instead, it will consist of kick-ass producers. Yes, while there may be fewer of us under age 65 per capita to pay for the costs of retirees and the very old, we will each have more than enough resources to cover these burdens. And there will be almost double the number of us in our prime years. While the exact mechanisms of sharing these burdens may certainly become the source of fierce political battles, that will be a mere sideshow compared to the larger changes.

Longevity is not the problem: It is the cure. Longevity is the Next Disruptor™.

4. We will all need to make an emotional as well as a biological shift. As we redefine our notion of longevity, it's one thing to consider bionic cells and circulatory systems, and other bodily functions. But there will also be other factors that will challenge our paradigms about aging. What will retirement look like? Will there even be "retirement" in the traditional sense? Or will there be a new system of careers—early, middle, and late? What will family structure look like? Will there be more blended and later-age new families?

And as we consider the many biological factors that affect aging—DNA, epigenetic switches, embryonic cells, and other ways of making yourself substantially younger—it's important to remember that relationships and connections will continue to play a major role in how well we age.[12] [13] [14] [15] In discussions of the future, the role of tech and medical advances can obscure what's most important—and what is the key to happiness and health:

We're human, and we're made to connect with other humans.

And that's why we want to live as long—and as young and vibrantly—as possible.

5. *Your posse and purpose will matter, too.* Just because the science of aging is advancing so fast doesn't mean that you should rule out other, "softer" factors when it comes to their influence on your health and longevity. Social connections and developing passions in life will also have an effect on how well and how long you live.

And while they may not dominate the headlines in the same way as stem cells and robotic cameras, social connections are worth thinking about as you consider how aging will change your life. We spend time later in the book looking at these psychological, emotional, and social factors, as they do change the way your brain and body work.

CHAPTER 2

YOUR FUTURE BODY, OUR FUTURE WORLD

Our predictions for what the world will look like by 2050

Years ago, we could never have predicted that one day you would wear on your wrist a computer more powerful than the room-filling IBM 360s of the 1960s.[1] We never could have predicted that you'd have thousands of entertainment-viewing options available on demand or could make bodily organs with a 3D printer. So how can we imagine what life will look like in another 30 years? Some changes are so rapid—so exponential—that they're hard to envision. Will we be closer to a sci-fi way of living with robotic body parts and spaceship shuttles? Will every heartbeat be analyzed instantly? Will phones be implanted in our ears? Will such fantasies become reality?

It's tempting to think that we'll be flying around in personal helicopters, all work will be carried out by robots, all disease will be eradicated, vaccines against potentially pandemic viruses will be able to be stockpiled and ready for widespread distribution within a day, and everyone will be healthy with statuesque bodies. But it's highly unlikely. People will still have self-doubts, overeat, succumb to the temptation of alcohol abuse and drugs, get insufficient exercise, suffer the effects of unmanaged stress, and not be safe enough. That is, bad choices will probably still abound.

Human behavior is difficult to predict; we have long known the damage that can be caused by alcohol abuse, obesity, smoking, drugs, and other threats to longevity. But many of these will be resolved, just as polio, mumps, measles, SARS, SARS-CoV-2 (we hope), and many other infectious diseases have been largely solved over the past hundred years

This means we are at a critical decision point in our country: to become healthier and to stay healthier, or to become sicker, burdened by managing preventable, lifestyle-induced chronic disease, or the consequences that these comorbidities cause. Those who choose the former will gain longer and more rewarding, fun-filled, and fulfilling lives.

As we look to the future, we're not going to speculate about flying cars or supersonic elevators or other sci-fi fantasies. Instead, we're going to take our best guess at what life will look like in three decades, based on projections backed by data, trends, and the best evidence currently available.

The Population Will Surge Despite Slower Birth Rates

The U.S. population will grow by 117.5 million people—a 1.05 percent annual growth rate—even as birth rates continue to decline. (Many other developed countries will have declining populations.) There will be approximately 2.2 people per household as single-member households continue to grow and living in group settings increases. Even as you may be reading reports about population declines, we anticipate great population growth with longer and healthier lives over the next 30 years.

One-Quarter of the U.S. Population Will Be Over 76

With the Great Age Reboot, you will begin to see dramatic shifts in the way the population looks (see the chart on page 28). The vast majority of the roughly 45 million Americans in their 30s today will still be alive in 2050—plus an additional million people will have been added to this cohort by net immigration over the next 30 years. Similarly, of those people currently in their 60s, about 74 percent (including net immigrants) will be alive in their 90s. Of the roughly 2.3 million alive today who are 90 years or older, as many as a quarter million (including immigrants in this age category) could still be alive at 120 years or more.

Whereas today 38 percent of the people we encounter are under the age of 30, less than 30 percent will be below age 30 in the year 2050. On the flip side, while today only about 11 percent are older than age 70, in the year 2050 we expect that fully 26 percent of the population will be over the age of 70. This means that chronologic youth will become relatively scarce, while agedness will become commonplace. This raises the question of whether there will be enough young, entry-level workers to satisfy the needs of an increasingly aged economy. It also highlights the fact that our larger economic structure will continue to evolve, with entry-level workers receiving unexpected earnings boosts due to their relative scarcity.

As these demographic shifts continue to unfold, so will consumption trends. By the year 2050, the consumption desires of those over age 70 will swamp those under age 30; as a result, the 70-plus crowd will experience unprecedented increases in their consumption behavior and political power and will have the physical capacity to take advantage of their financial resources. (One suspects that their purchasing desires will have more in common with those in their 50s today than with those currently in their 70s and 80s.) Therefore, while travel outlays and expenditures for retirement communities will certainly rise, this increase may be far less than one might expect, as many older people will still be actively employed. Plastic surgery practices and genetic skin rebooting will no doubt thrive. Rebooted age creates rebooted spending patterns and rebooted retailers to serve them.

We Will Experience Another Housing Boom

As the benefits of rebooting set in and the aging population increases annually, housing will need to rise to nearly two million new units a year. This will create a housing stock roughly 40 percent larger than today's 140 million units, skewed to both the younger demographic and the 90-plus demographic. As people remain healthier and live longer, they will work longer. This means that they will remain in their homes seven or more years longer before deciding whether to move closer to sun and warmth or to retire near their roots. While many will move upon retirement, even more will remain in place, or near their current residence, for connectivity with their healthy friends and family. The desire for rich, full, meaningful social lives will thus fuel growth not only in the Sun Belt, but also in the current major cities. We suspect that new single-family homes will have fewer bedrooms, but larger rooms and greater amenities.

We also can envision a world with different living arrangements: more multi-"family" homes. The abodes of the future, we predict, will feature larger bedrooms and bathrooms, and smaller personal living areas for six to 12 people—many people will choose to spend most of their time in the jointly owned and shared common spaces that come with recreation, dining, education, daycare, and more. In addition, the "renting" of shared environments will become more prevalent (especially among older people and in Sun Belt communities).

New Educational Models Will Inspire Fourth Careers

Education will be completed before age 30. But the urgency to finish by age 18 or 22 or 27 (depending on whether your goal is to complete high school, college, trade school, or post-doctoral work) will be lessened by longer life expectancy. (There will also be more "gap" years and experiences for the young funded by their wealthier and healthier grandparents.) While we suspect that few 50-year-olds will be willing to uproot to "go back to campus," they will nevertheless need to learn new skills. Though successful online learning has thus far been spotty, it's safe to assume that rigorous virtual training programs will probably evolve. And while it might make for a cute movie plot, we do not expect an explosion in serious learning by the rebooted population over 70. Education is not always appealing for older people. But there will certainly be reeducation for second, third, and maybe fourth careers . . . so educators will need to figure out how to make that process fun.

Virtual Medicine Will Be the Standard

We picture a world in which many of your medical issues will be handled on a virtual basis. Monitors on your body will be connected to medical facilities able to diagnose and treat a variety of ailments and issues. It will be a personal, customized experience with a nearly immediate response time. That could mean immediate treatment for heart attacks or immediate detection of cancer before it becomes sizable. But food, physical activity, stress management, friends, passions, and other beneficial choices will still be within your control.

Plastic Surgery Will Benefit From the Reboot

This is a sector that will experience explosive growth over the next 30 years. If I feel 40, I will want to act and look 40, using the financial resources of a 70-year-old. Face-lifts, nips and tucks, injections, creams, and high-tech fitness centers to improve body shape and complement plastic surgery will abound.

Most of Us Will Have a Higher Standard of Living

Based on historic growth rates, real GDP per household will be approximately 55 percent higher than today, meaning that unimaginable additional consumer and societal purchasing power will exist. Just think what we could do today if every person had 55 percent more spending power. Moreover, rebooting health will free up more than $800 billion to spend on other things, as the burdens of chronic diseases are rebooted out of existence. Ten percent of the savings from rebooted health comes out to $1,600 per person. The economy will be booming because of reduced medical costs and the amazing productivity derived from a longer working age—i.e., human capital.

But Not Everyone Will

The inequalities in health and wealth could be larger than ever, due to the compounding effect of extra years on both health and savings accounts and with bad decisions driving the inequities even further.[2] Those not adopting healthier lifestyles will experience more chronic disease, while the rest will attain higher levels of health. This will not only allow greater earning years for the healthy, but that greater income will mean more savings. And those who save wisely will be saving for more years, allowing the "magic" of compounding to raise wealth levels of long-working healthy savers to unimaginable levels.

The good news is that society's resources will be massively increased, and wise, healthy savers will be able to enjoy comfortable, long lives. The bad news is that the inevitable resulting inequities will threaten to create an "us/them" mindset. This possibility increases the relevance of forced savings programs, currently employed in Australia and several other countries (and recently passed in the U.S. House of Representatives with overwhelming bipartisan support), to help minimize financial inequality. We believe such programs will come to America (and the rest of the world too), and will help social inequality decrease as longevity and prime years increase. The challenge that faces such forced savings programs is that the political left does not support them, as they believe "society" should support people's retirement, while the political right believes that people should not be compelled to save. The result is that highly effective mandatory savings plans have not garnered notable support. While we have some sympathy for both arguments, we believe that mandatory retirement savings programs would be beneficial because they overcome the lack of discipline and financial

DEMOGRAPHIC DIFFERENCES

As society changes, so will attitudes and approaches based on your age and stage. Some of our related predictions:

Those in Their 30s in 2050	In the year 2050, the major concerns facing those in their 30s will still be very similar to those of their peers today: finding a mate, starting a family, nurturing a career, seeking work/life balance, and developing deeper relationships with friends and beloved family members (many of whom will not be blood family). They will still work, they will still pay taxes, they will still find joy and frustration in dealing with their ever extending families. Their children will be subject to fewer diseases and experience more robust health than any previous young generation; their parents will not only benefit from improved traditional medical advances but will also be using genetic reboots to reduce the toll of chronic diseases.
Those in Their 60s and 70s in 2050	About 60 to 70 percent of this demographic cohort will remain in the workforce as they realize that longer, healthier lives will require a longer financial runway. Their children and grandchildren will be the healthiest population in history. Those in their 60s and 70s will have benefited from 15 to 30 years of genetic reboot technology, from transforming scarred heart tissue into coordinated contracting heart muscle cells to massively reducing the incidence and severity of chronic disease. Genetic engineering may even allow the ravages associated with smoking, drugs, and alcohol to be greatly reduced if not reversed. This group will not only have the wisdom of their age; they will have the health and physical vitality of 35-year-olds today. Their youthful years will increase.
Those in Their 90s and 100s in 2050	When today's boomers, currently aged up to 75, reach the 100-year-old range, some will still be working, and some will be as healthy as are today's 50- to 65-year-olds. They will have greater wealth to help support their lifestyles, and their greater health, derived from genetically engineered reboots, will free up considerable financial resources. In their 90s, a few will still be enjoying relationships with their parents and some will be caring for parents approaching their 120th birthdays. The improved health and mobility of this cohort will allow them the opportunity to lead more active lives and enjoy their children, grandchildren, great-grandchildren, and even great-greats. Many will pursue new careers or start new businesses.

sophistication that plagues many citizens. But we admit that it is a politically challenged proposition.

Rebooted health is the solution for the federal budget deficit created during the late 2010s and early 2020s due to significantly increased spending, tax law changes, and pandemic relief, because it will significantly reduce the needed financial outlays for veterans, government employees, and Medicaid/Medicare recipients (the costs per person will be reduced because care can be delayed as people are healthy longer).

And as people live longer and healthier lives, particularly without the complications of chronic disease, medical outlay growth will notably lag GDP growth. In practice, this means that the feared explosion of the federal deficit due to aging citizens will never come to pass; spending on health care for the elderly will be delayed by at least 20 years and that money can be channeled into pension retirement programs and other productive activities. Improved health means that money that would be spent on medical care when we are 50, 60, and 70 will not be necessary for 20 to 30 extra years. This money will be both invested and spent on nonmedical choices (leisure, housing, education, technology, etc.).

As to the accumulated U.S. federal deficits of today, they are only about 20 percent of the current net wealth of U.S. citizens. That is, our society is a net donor to future generations. To put the current $24 trillion federal debt in some context, it amounts to only about one year of GDP. More important, it is dwarfed by our $120 trillion in household wealth. This means we could pay it off with one year of income or pay it off with our assets and have $96 trillion in tangible wealth remaining. Further, since the present value of the U.S. economy (current wealth plus the future value of GDP) is roughly $800 trillion, the current federal debt is a mere 3 percent of the present value of our economy. It is not a matter of whether we can afford it, but rather the far more difficult political question of who will pay. And as has always been the case, most people will want others to pay. Rebooting will not change human nature.

We will also see the demise of defined benefit pension programs, and a complete shift to defined contribution programs. This will increase savings for workers, providing greater financial security. As has always been the case, the elderly will probably experience less luxurious retirements than they envision, even as they live far better lives than any previous retired generation. This will no doubt be aided by the inheritance many of today's boomers will receive as the generation before them dies.

PART 2

SEDUCTIVE SCIENCE

A look at the major medical advances that are coming soon—and coming fast

Today, it's common to read about such futuristic phenomena as driverless cars and hotels on the moon—which is why although the contents of the next chapters may not seem shocking, they could also easily be dismissed as whimsy. Why? The era of the bionic woman and man is finally upon us. Support on the federal level (most support starts there) for research into the mechanisms of aging is growing. It increased from $1.807 billion in 2012 to $3.738 billion in 2020.[1] And there is a much greater increase when other funding source increases are included. The number of patents related to longevity increased more than 400 percent from 2009 to 2014 and quadrupled again from 2014 to 2019.[2]

Combining medicine, biology, and engineering, the trio of the National Institute on Aging, private foundations, and pharma-supported longevity scientists is building better and more resilient bodies. This research is happening all over the world—with a special eye toward looking at how to engineer our bodies to work better, repair damage, and ultimately stay youthful longer.

The entire process begins with cells, the building blocks of our bodies. Each one of us has trillions, which contain our DNA; our DNA holds the genetic information that controls the way our bodies function (and determines our similarities to and differences from each other).

There are many different kinds of cells—nerve cells, skin cells, white blood cells, all kinds—serving different purposes, depending on their biological location and assignment. The mitochondria, or power plants, of each of these different types of cells, convert food into energy to help your body function properly.

As you might imagine with such a complex biological infrastructure, a zillion and three things can go wrong. Cells can be infected by a virus or bacteria. They can be attacked by enemy toxins and transformed, as with cancer. Or they can simply wear out and wear down over time, as is the case in most aging-related problems (sort of as if your body has rusted out). In many instances, our medical advances have worked to help eradicate these problems.

Today's advances are where things get exciting. Researchers now are focused on advancements that affect cells in two different ways: rejuvenation and regeneration.[3] Here's how they work in broad terms.

Rejuvenation: These advances slow the aging process by helping bodily systems "act" younger. You can go through a process that has an effect on the infrastructure, just like a massage may loosen up sore muscles or an oil change peps up an engine. Those procedures may not actually give you a new muscle or a new engine, but they prolong and improve performance of the existing system by slowing down the aging process.

That process can happen at the cellular level, too. With certain procedures or treatments, cells can get their metaphorical massage or oil change to extend the life span of their effectiveness. And this rejuvenation directly slows aging, because the cells can "act" younger for longer.

Regeneration: What's better than having cells act younger? Having them actually *be* younger. This is what we mean by cellular regeneration. What if scientists could actually change cells, change mitochondria, and change the switches that control your DNA so that you have your original factory settings back again—and they are set to "younger"? That's what's happening right now in mice and dog models, where a manipulation can change aging cells to youthful ones.

But this process is about more than just slow aging or healthy aging. New research advances into aging mechanisms make us believe longevity is about to take a big leap. These are some of the more prominent (of many) that may affect aging in the future:

- Stem cell production without immunogenicity
- Autophagy with intermittent fasting
- Senolytics, including therapeutic plasma exchange
- Gene editing
- Induced tissue regeneration
- Epigenetic reboot

- Elimination of obesity, specifically in regard to white-to-brown fat transformation
- Immunotherapy and immunologic targeting
- Hormetic hyperbaric oxygen therapy
- Photodynamic and energy therapies
- Mitochondrial restoration
- Microbiome reprogramming
- Bionic bodies
- Proteostasis

The metaphor here is getting a new engine in a car or new pipes in a house—not just for individual organs, but for your whole body. Changing the switches that govern the guts of the machine can make the actual machine live on for a much longer time, because it's not about getting the most miles out of the original engine; it's actually getting a new engine. When this process is achieved, it will turn our linear life span increases into exponential ones.

The next few chapters will take you through the advances that we believe have the most potential for changing the way we live and the way our bodies will work.

CHAPTER 3

THE CELLULAR CHAMELEONS

Why stem cells are one of our greatest hopes for a longer and healthier life

People who develop heart failure after a series of heart attacks live in a tough spot: They can't exercise, they must lower their sodium intake, and they must watch their diets carefully, more than they normally might do.

What happens if they don't follow these guidelines? They'll end up in the ER (or worse) because they've lost the heart cells that can effectively pump blood. The disease has destroyed those heart cells and replaced them with fibrous tissue, or the heart cells have become unable to contract due to damage, and those cells can cause their neighboring, still normal cells to pump a little out of sequence and thus inefficiently. The heart is damaged, and the effect is profound: Breathing is a struggle—if not damn near impossible—because the lungs fill with fluid.

The life expectancy for those at this stage of heart failure hovers around 18 months, and these are unhealthy months.[1]

In January 2020, physicians at Osaka University in Japan performed the world's first transplant of a special kind of cardiac muscle stem cells. The patient was part of a study seeking to save cardiac patients from their death sentence.[2]

Stem cells are the matriarch of the human body: the cells from which all other cells are derived. Your specialized cells—heart, brain, and all others—come from your stem cells.

The scientists in the study used a certain class of stem cells called iPSCs—induced pluripotent stem cells. These are cells that the researchers harvested from older cells and regressed back into stem cells, which then have the ability to self-renew by dividing and developing. Using Nobel Prize–winning technology (also developed in Japan), the scientists harvested iPSCs from donor tissues, returned them to their immature state, and then placed them in a human body. The cells could then develop into any cell type and help with repairing damaged cells. Implanted in the heart, they could release chemicals that help form healthy vessels and improve cardiac function.

In the experiment, 20 to 25 million young, healthy, strong cells were microsurgically implanted into the research subjects' damaged, failing hearts.

The scientists programmed and cultured the stem cells to produce infant heart cells. These heart cells were amazing because they had no immune markers that would cause rejection.

In six weeks, those cells replaced the function and actually recycled the proteins from the poorly functioning cells.

After six months, early indications in the first two patients showed that the technique was working—essentially reversing the damage and restoring the heart to youthful function.

Now, let's be clear that we don't know if the treatment will work in everyone or for how long. Will these stem cells become heart cells? Will they synchronize with neighboring cells? Will this process work with all causes of heart failure?

The answers remain unclear, but the hope is that this stem-cell rejuvenation can extend life expectancy not by months, but by years—more than 20 years.

Some medical scientists think that by 2030, we'll be able to use this replacement process with any organ or tissue or structure except maybe your brain. (Though it could apply to parts of your brain, too: In late 2020, researchers from a variety of entities, including the University of Barcelona, developed neurons from stem cells that could be injected into the brain.[3 4]) This is the world we're living in—one in which a death sentence can be turned into a life extension—a life extension with the energy you had 30 years ago.

And that is the promise—the hope—of medical advances revolving around stem cells.

| | | | | |

We like to think of a stem cell sort of like a master of impressions, a comedian who can mimic a thousand voices. That's because the very nature of the initial (or embryonic) stem cell is that it can turn into any other cell in the body. Now scientists can take stem cells that are a little more developed and specialized to one type of tissue and regress them to the way they were when you were only an eight-cell organism. These cells, which are able to develop into any—or at least many—types of tissues, are known as "pluripotent" cells. They can get rid of their trait that would reject the cells (called immunogenicity) so they can go from one human to many, and transform into specific tissues like heart, liver, or kidney cells.[5]

Stem cells are chameleons that can adapt to whatever situation is needed. That much we know, but we haven't yet figured out how we get stem cells to do the job of reversing the entire cellular clock—to not only make a heart that is 30 years younger, but to make all of your parts 30 years younger.

So far, it appears that those methods could come from two directions.

One, you could harvest your own stem cells. Taken from your own blood marrow, stem cells could be grown in culture as a certain type of cell, then injected into problem areas to grow into cells that form new and healthy tissue. There are a couple of problems with going in this direction. Not only does your body appear to have a finite number of stem cells that can be produced over the course of a lifetime, but also it currently takes a long time for a harvested stem cell to develop into the cell marked for another part of the tissue (approximately three weeks but getting shorter all the time).

Two, you could receive healthy stem cells from a donor. That would mean that your body could accept donor stem cells that would be healthy and injected into the problem areas. The possibilities are limitless. Have a problem with your heart, lungs, a knee, or anything else? Well, just order up a mass-produced dose of stem cells to clear damaged tissue and replace it with healthy kinds. Sound too good to be true? It is for now. That's because the big roadblock revolves around immunity. It's not enough for stem cells to do their job of being new and young. They also have to be accepted by your body—your body can't perceive those cells as foreign invaders and want to reject them. In addition, there have to be enough cells to effectively heal a problem—and those stem-cell counts could be in the 100 million range for each body area that needs attention (small animals need 10 to 30 million stem cells to regrow heart tissue or cartilage). That's a lot of cells to develop, mass-produce, and have available (all with the ability to circumvent the body's natural immune-rejection process).

Yet that is what researchers from across the world are working on rigorously—to see if we can leverage the character-istics of these impressionist-like cells to heal damaged and aging body parts.

||||||

Let's take a step back and see the science in action: Your native stem cells are the ones from which all other cells—blood, brain, and more—are derived. And stem cells can also become new stem cells, by dividing and propagating.

Here's another way that stem cells are maternal: They come in and fix things. But instead of doing so with a hug or a kernel of wisdom, they achieve their ends by repairing damage in the body, replacing damaged cells or growing into new ones. In fact, this is how virtually all parts of your body heal.

When you scrape your knee or have a sunburn, it's not cells from neighboring skin that come to the rescue. It's stem cells (assuming your blood supply is healthy and intact). Same goes for when you have a heart attack, infection, or other inter-nal threat.

The proteins that nourish stem cells, called exosomes,

foster growth and help the stem cells develop into a new version of whatever is needed: heart muscle, skin, brain, what have you.[6] One key: You need healthy blood flow to make this work, because that's how the messages travel from the heart or brain, telling stem cells where to go. We learned how important blood flow was in relation to stem cells from a female heart transplanted into a male patient.[7] If that female heart then had a heart attack, after which blood flow was restored quickly enough, the heart would repair itself with male stem cells, which would become new contracting heart muscle cells over six weeks. Yes, it initially was a bad heart with a low ability to send blood to the rest of the body, but over the course of six weeks that bad female heart grew new heart muscle cells from the repairing stem cells of the man's body and generated a lot of blood flow.

While we used to think stem cells were immortal, that's not the case. Researchers have found that they're preprogrammed to live for only 40 to 60 duplications (called the Hayflick limit).[8] (One indication that you are near death is that your stem cells have too short an end—called a telomere—to

Breakthrough Bonus

One recent study found that when older people breathed oxygen through a mask in a hyperbaric chamber (for 90 minutes five days a week), they lengthened their telomeres by a significant 20 percent; this is important because telomeres are related to overall age deterioration. The longer they are, the longer you live.[9] Another bonus: The study participants also reduced cells that can become inflamed and weaken the immune system—another marker for aging. This study needs replication to be validated. But pay attention to the media or our GreatAgeReboot.com website for an update, as such replication attempts are already in progress.

duplicate.) So, to repair ourselves again and again for youthful longevity, we will need to replenish our supply of stem cells.

And here's another hurdle: If too many stem cells are asked to regenerate tissue, that increases the chance that some of them will divide endlessly and become cancerous.

| | | | | |

We are seeing some success and advances in the stem-cell field. For instance, researchers and neurosurgeons at Stanford University took 18 people who for more than five years had been missing some of their brain area that controlled motor function and injected stem cells into the areas of the brain that needed to be restored. In seven of the 18 people, they reported a significant amount of motor function returned, indicating that stem cells served a repairing function. (Apparently, when the patients suffered their original stroke or brain damage, blood flow wasn't restored fast enough for their own stem cells to repair their brains at the time, or they didn't have enough stem cells to make the repair.)[10]

So one theory is that if we can generate more stem cells combined with their exosomal growth factors, we can improve our body's repair processes.[11]

Some research indicates that intermittent calorie restriction can help. When people were put on a specific low-protein, low-simple-carb diet of about 1,000 calories on day one and 750 calories for the next four days, then went back to a Mediterranean-style diet, Valter Longo and his team at the University of Southern California found substantial growth in some components of stem cells.[12] [13] Interesting note: This was an accidental discovery; workers in the lab fed calorie-restricted animals by mistake. Instead of throwing the data out, Longo wanted to see what would happen with restriction and refeeding. It had never been done before, as it was thought that calorie restriction had to be forever. But calorie restriction and refeeding generated more stem cells, able to rejuvenate any area of the body that needs repair.

Even finding that calorie restriction alone extended life was an accidental discovery. In 1933, during the Great Depression, scientist Clive McCay at Cornell University wanted to keep his lab going but didn't have enough money for food for all the animals. So he made half of them go on a 35 percent calorie restriction diet. The mice that were forced on calorie restriction lived 30 percent longer than the fully fed group.[14]

At this point, rejuvenating areas of your body with stem cells grown in culture looks to be a body-specific solution—that is, stem cells can target one area, like the heart pumping cells, or cartilage in a joint, or a bone, rather than refresh your entire body and systems.

You may know people who have gotten a "stem cell treatment." In the United States, stem cell clinics (then generating over $3 billion in revenue) were told to cease to exist by April 2020, and the Food and Drug Administration (FDA) has long warned people about promises made by clinics because they are likely to be unsubstantiated and potentially harmful.

These clinics have allure for people in pain—say, from sore or arthritic knees. Patients go to a clinic and receive an injection of platelet-rich plasma (PRP) and their own stem cells (harvested via bone marrow) and perhaps get temporary relief. The problem? The number of stem cells is usually minuscule—

say, a couple of hundred cells compared with the tens of millions needed for true rejuvenation. But injections of PRP can reduce inflammation—and thus, pain.[15] Because the patients then feel better, that gave them the impression that the stem cells must be working. Or it could have been that the patients may have been getting better all along, and the timing of the injection just made it seem like it had had an effect.

The relief patients feel often comes from the decrease in inflammation—which is almost always only temporary (unless you are lucky enough to get a senolytic effect—see Chapter 4). So "stem cell" treatments are usually supplying only a wallet biopsy: The companies giving them are taking a sample of their patients' money—and quite a large one at that, at several thousands of dollars per treatment.

The real hope for long-term antiaging remedies from stem cells, however, is what's on the horizon—harvesting or donating stem cells to heal and rejuvenate damaged cells with the quantity needed to do so. Long-term repair, as opposed to temporary relief.

Breakthrough Bonus

One of the challenges of getting blood stem cells to help with longevity: You need a lot of them, and a specific kind (called hematopoietic stem cells), which can be scarce. Researchers at the Centre for Genomic Regulation in Barcelona and at Columbia University have identified a protein that could help with growing a lot of these stem cells (not just inside the body, but outside as well).[16] These blood stem cells could help treat cancers, autoimmune problems, and more. Fun fact: The researchers used an algorithm to identify proteins that could reprogram some blood cells into a specific kind of cell.

| CHAPTER 4 |

CELLULAR MAGIC TRICKS

The longevity promise of reengineering your aging cells

I t sounds like a scene from a Tom Hanks movie: Buddy grows old, Buddy doesn't like it, Buddy wants to slow down and stop the clock. So Buddy bargains with a wizard who promises a youth potion. Drink this, the wizard says, and you will be young again. Buddy obliges. *Gulp gulp gulp gulp.* "Abracadabra, make aging disappear." And with that, Buddy is young again: Gray hair is gone, posture is upright, muscles are strong, fat is zapped, disease is nowhere to be found. The once-old is the now-young. The magic potion was able to take away the old cells and recycle them into young cells.

In a way, this was happening in Mayo Clinic labs in the early 2010s.[1] Scientists there were using a genetic technique to remove old cells, improving or removing age-related diseases from mice. But, like just about anything when it comes to medical advances, it's one thing to show something in mice and/or rats, and another to replicate it in humans. That leap is often Grand Canyon–wide—and where many medical advances die a disappointing death. After all, orange juice in the right quantities can cause some cancers in mice and cure other cancers in mice, so you can't just forecast an effect in humans because the technique or therapy works in mice or rats.

Yet in May 2020, news came out that Unity Biotechnology—a Mayo offshoot, under the leadership of Ned David and Judith Campisi—was using the same technology and approach in phase I and now phase II drug trials in human volunteers.[2] (While the phase II trial failed, the success seen in phase I has encouraged the company to continue its research.)

Here's what they did: In a small study of people with pain from MRI-documented osteoarthritis, their drug or a placebo was injected into the knee. The 12 patients in the highest dose groups reported that, unlike for those who received the placebo, the drug took away over 80 percent of pain and restored at least 80 percent of function for at least three months.

The pain, inflammation, and osteoarthritis largely disappeared.

Although this was a very small sample, the results were pretty astounding—especially for a condition that is primarily chalked up as an inevitable part of aging. Your knee gets arthritis as you lose cartilage and cushioning, you bear the pain until you can't stand it anymore, and in the developed world you then get a knee replacement. The disease ultimately wins, and we humans counteract by constructing new, artificial knees. They work well, yes, but they're not your original parts and you have to go through surgery and often difficult rehab to restore even some function, let alone 80 percent of normal. But the promise of eliminating the pain with one shot? Slowing the clock and keeping our original parts? It sure does have a "step-right-up" carnival-barker allure to it. A potion of youth indeed.

Now, this drug failed in phase II trials. But other approaches in this category are being tested with some promising early results in humans. In any case, this is a story not just about knees and rats, but about potential: What happens if this same drug and same approach could be applied to many parts and systems of your body?

Make your heart as good as new? Your brain? Your back? Every other part of your body that ages?

That's the promise of what lies ahead with one of the major players in the longevity race: senolytics. "Senescence" means the "process of growing old," while "lytics" means "anti." Senolytics is anti–growing old.

The senolytic hypothesis of age reversal has been worked on with increasing intensity and dollars since 2008. The basic mission: to use senolytic agents to harvest old and damaged cells—called senescent or senile cells—to slow down aging processes. For example, scientists from the University of California, San Francisco, continuously infused the blood of young mice into old mice—and found that the old mice functioned as young ones.[3] One of the effects was that the number of stem cells and their growth factors in the old mice increased.

The theory is that senile cells hang around in bodies, increasing in numbers and effects as we age, and cause a whole lot of destruction. (They actually are formed even when we are infants but are recycled by our bodies and do not start accumulating until we are near age 30.) They contribute to inflammation, and, in what is even more destructive, they secrete substances that turn neighboring healthy cells senescent.[4]

You know the saying that you're only as good as the friends you hang around with? These senescent cells are the bad influences. They turn strong cells old. Another way to think about it is to look at the way a piece of fruit goes bad. It starts with one small rotting area, but then that rot spreads to other areas, and then to neighboring pieces of fruit, until the whole fruit bowl and all neighboring pieces of fruit have brown, deteriorating flesh.

This is why senolytics is so promising: It works by getting rid of these hooligan cells that turn healthy cells to the dark side.

The effect felt profound and optimistic when a group of researchers from the Mayo Clinic showed research in rodents using this advance. They revealed a photo of two elderly rodents, both the same age, from the same litter. The one that had aged naturally was shrunken and looked old, while the counterpart that had had the senolytic treatment had the pep of a high school cheerleader. You could *see* the difference from the outside—and that's not even counting the changes that occurred on the inside.

Other researchers have reported that treatment with seno-lytics changes the blood so much that the older rats getting the blood of young rats essentially morph from 109-week-old rats to 30-week-old rats.[5]

What makes the knee experiment by Unity Biotechnology so interesting, then, is that this was the first report of a drug injected into a specific site in humans where the old cells were harvested and the surrounding cells became less inflamed— and with just one shot. The pain largely disappeared, and the inflammation disappeared (we do not know if more joint car-tilage actually was created).

Today, there are promising experiments being done on all sorts of body parts when it comes to senolytics.

For example, a senolytic combo has been found to restore vision in animals with induced wet macular degeneration—the most common form of vision loss in aging humans.[6] Mice that were the equivalent of an elderly human have regained their younger vision. Imagine stopping sight loss with a senolytic when you are 85, and then reprogramming your eyes and eye muscles so your eyesight can be as good as it was when you were 20.

Another experiment showed that senolytic agents restored hydration into the disks of the spine; that hydration is important for proper spine functioning and to avoid and reduce back pain (one of the major sources of pain in this country and one of the primary reasons for doctor visits and missed work).[7]

But the implications of what senolytics can do to the heart and brain are where the most excitement lies.

Your heart's pumping cells need to work in concert with all other heart pumping cells to most efficiently move blood throughout the body. As you age and your cells become old, that timing can be off.

If your heart muscle cells do not contract and relax with perfect timing, you don't pump blood efficiently. It's like two pianists in a duet just one second off in hitting their notes. The concert sounds lousy. With heart cells, that slight change in timing means you develop heart failure and your lungs fill up with fluid.[8]

When you have weakened blood flow, your body is less able to function efficiently. When you're tired after a meal, for example, that's because your blood is being used for digestion, so it's less able to pump blood throughout the rest of your body. This happens more frequently when we're older due to the damage over time to the blood flow system. So senolytics offer the promise of overall improvement and function of the heart by restoring youthful function to the cells that make it work.

Two drugs approved for other uses appear, in studies by Mayo Clinic researchers, to have a senolytic effect—they combine to harvest and get rid of old cells to allow neighboring cells to return to normal function and improve the blood pumping done by your heart.[9] And more efficient senolytics are being studied. In some research on heart attacks in mice, scientists found that those treated with senolytics recovered 35 percent more cardiac function and lived 20 percent longer than those without the treatment.[10]

This is where much research is headed:

How do we change cellular structures, processes, and functioning to flip the switch on aging and disease? A related area of research involves the cellular process called autophagy.

This process has been gaining more mainstream visibility as more people understand its role. A very complex process, autophagy is sort of a recycling of your body.[11] It helps your body clean up and repair itself by churning up damaged cells and getting rid of (eating) the unwanted cell parts while keeping the cells intact (the word "autophagy" means "self-eating").

Now, our bodies are not constantly in a state of autophagy. It turns on and off. Recent research shows that we can have some control over it, inducing the process by periodically fasting.[12] There also is quite a bit of evidence that autophagy helps us slow aging by quieting inflammation and helping build our immune system. Clean out the cellular trash, reap the longevity benefits.

But this is where things get tricky. Researchers are looking at the role that autophagy plays in cancer. Some evidence shows that autophagy may protect cancer at one stage and thereby help tumors that have been damaged by chemotherapy regrow. Makes sense, right? If autophagy is responsible for renewing injured cells, then the process could also repair cancer cells damaged by chemotherapy. Autophagy could be cancer's best friend.

Now, science is showing that altering autophagy may have a role in influencing the growth of cancer, making it a fertile area for drug development. That's why we'll be seeing autophagy inhibitors—drugs that can stop the autophagy process and potentially stop the growth of tumors. That has many implications when it comes to longevity—if you can figure out how to stop cancer from growing, you will increase the chances of extending life.[13]

Much of the work of Eileen White, of Rutgers University, has revolved around autophagy inhibitors that kill cancer— working by inhibiting autophagy so that cancers can't hide out in the body and renew themselves, which allows other cancer treatments to more effectively kill them.[14] So you may not want to institute a fasting process during chemotherapy as that fasting could induce autophagy and allow your cancer to hibernate and then return stronger. However, after cancer, you do want to try intermittent fasting or time-restricted feeding, as early data imply that these simple, side-effect-free, no-medication-involved practices can help you regain impaired functions and experience better quality of life as a cancer survivor.

Breakthrough Bonus

Researchers from the University of California at Berkeley found that a process called a plasma exchange could work to slow aging by lowering pro-inflammatory proteins that tend to increase with age.[15] The already FDA-approved process rejuvenates muscle and brain cells. It could have an effect similar to that of senolytics, acting like a switch to help old cells turn young. Studies have shown that plasma exchange in humans with Alzheimer's could help slow cognitive decline by 50 percent. That is a wow-wow-wow.

One of the big challenges in studying aging is this: Aging isn't a disease that has an end point. Ultimately, death is the end point, but aging is really a cluster of diseases, processes, conditions, and system errors that result in loss of years and loss of quality of life.

But to study any treatment, you need a specific end point or marker of success or failure. That's why treatments like senolytics are studied in conditions like knee arthritis or back pain, or stem cells in heart failure patients; you can measure results in tangible, specific outcomes.[16] You can't measure a death point of one person because there's no way of knowing precisely what the alternative death point would have been with or without the treatment. And to study death for a population, you would have to wait and see if that drug, or treatment, or lifestyle change, like intermittent fasting, really affected the age at which people died—which would take more years than most scientists have.

So, for the time being, there will be some extrapolation happening—if senolytics can work in arthritis, could it be applied to overall aging? Could the senolytic drug that took away knee inflammation and pain be injected into the brain to prevent memory deterioration?

That is the promise of this treatment, which if it works, could be available after FDA approval sometime around 2026. And if you add in senolytic treatments for your back joints, knee joints, heart and lungs, or brain and eyes, you could be another 12 years younger before 2030.

Breakthrough Bonus

Targeted therapy for cancer can include more than chemotherapy or immunotherapy. New therapies can focus on a specific part of a cancer cell, such as a protein or gene that stimulates the cancer to grow or spread. This is the case for the breakthrough drug ibrutinib, which inhibits a specific enzyme in lymphocytic leukemia cells.

CHAPTER 5

YOUR DNA DESTINY, EDITED

DNA manipulation is the next frontier of genetic engineering and an epigenetic reboot

n the summer of 2020—while the world was in the midst of dealing with the COVID-19 pandemic—University of Virginia researchers made a discovery that could be an important piece of the puzzle in solving one of our deadliest forms of cancer.[1]

They found the gene responsible for at least some types of glioblastoma, an aggressive and nearly always fatal form of brain cancer. This oncogene (cancer-causing gene) is essential for the survival of this specific cancer. In glioblastoma, cancer cells latch on to the gene, proliferate, spread, and kill the person, usually very quickly. In experiments in mice, the UVA researchers were able to identify the gene specific to the glio tumor and block its activity. The effect? The cancer died and there was no damage to healthy cells.

While we're still a long way from determining whether any therapies involving this gene can successfully treat glioblastoma in humans, this research puts a spotlight on another promising frontier in longevity: gene therapy and gene editing.

This knowledge all stems from the Human Genome Project work that defined what makes you *you*. Four chemicals—represented by the four letters A, C, G, and T—come in base pairs to determine everything about you, from hair color to disease predisposition. Your individual sequence? About 3.2 billion letters in those 22,500 genes. That's your individual code. That code is housed in 23 pairs of chromosomes—one of each pair from each parent. Each chromosome contains hundreds to thousands of genes that contain code that directs the manufacture of proteins and controls cell growth, function, and survival.

As you know from the number of times you're asked for a family history, genetics influences your health. You may be predisposed to be male or female, or to get cancer or heart disease, or any other number of ailments, based on your heredity. But here's where things get interesting. Of those 22,500 DNA genes, only about 1,500 are "on" at any one time—suggesting that we do have biological on-off switches and suggesting that we could control about 80 percent of which genes are on or off by the lifestyle choices we make (like with diet and stress management).[2] These "epigenetic" switches have been the source of much discussion and confusion about our ability to control our genes. But many lifestyle behaviors have been identified as having influences over the switches. And remember, healthy cells re-create healthy cells, while unhealthy cells create more unhealthy cells.[3][4]

Now, why do we need to change which of your genes are on or off? Some may have defects that we were born with, or some of our DNA may have been damaged over time. As we age, our environment and our normal cellular processes cause damage to our genes and to their switches (the epigenes). This damage compounds over the course of one's life and is known to accelerate aging.

All cancers are caused by mutation of one or more genes. These mutations are usually acquired, but occasionally are inherited. More than 560 human cancer genes have been identified so far.[5] The most common cause of acquired cancer-causing gene mutation is random DNA "mistakes" during cell division. Other causes include smoking, aging, X-rays, ultra-violet radiation, radioactive materials, chemicals (e.g., Agent Orange, asbestos), hormones, obesity, and viruses.

So, gene errors as the major cause of cancer and some other diseases means there's a lot of potential for genetic fixes to get genes back to functioning normally. One of the more high-profile ways to do this comes from a method called CRISPR/Cas9.

CRISPR is the Nobel Prize–winning method that works like biological scissors: A virus vector is inserted into the body with a mission to detect the faulty genetic code. The virus vector with RNA and a protein finds the exact spot and the protein cuts it, essentially eliminating the code that is causing the faulty messages. Slice and destroy.[6] And the best part: The technology marks and remembers what it cuts so it can defend against any future developments or DNA mutations and eliminate or change them as well.

The method, so far, has been used to engineer solutions as diverse as increasing cocaine resistance in mice, reducing genetic deafness in mice, reversing a form of muscular dystrophy in dogs, reversing a form of heart failure in humans, and killing cancer cells in humans.[7] And there's hope that the technology could help with Alzheimer's and other brain-related diseases. Chinese researchers have reported using the technology to genetically engineer babies so their cells cannot easily replicate the HIV virus and thus have a much lower risk of developing AIDS.[8]

The possibilities here include being able to edit genes associated with depression, Alzheimer's, addiction, and arthritis, as well as other conditions that cause aging, poor health, and death. Society is already debating: Where do we draw the line in gene manipulation? Will parents be able to choose to turn off genes in newborns for certain characteristics that they don't like, that perhaps have nothing to do with health? For now, this does not deter us from studying the mechanism that can slow the aging process, but it will continue to be an important social discussion.

Over the years, breakthrough areas involving DNA have flipped scientific thinking on its head, in that we no longer have to believe that people are forever beholden to the genes they were born with. Instead, the promise of the future is that we will have the power to change the function of some genes or eliminate genes that can damage us. We may be able to essentially change our medical futures with a biological delete button.

We are seeing this play out in humans in some cases. For example, gene therapy is in human trials to treat sickle cell disease,[9] a blood disorder prevalent in the African American community. In the disease, a gene mutation changes the shape of red blood cells and inhibits oxygen from passing from those red cells to parts of the body. But with gene therapy, that gene can be blocked to allow more production of near-normal or normal red blood cells that carry oxygen to tissues. This is gene editing—eliminating a specific gene so an abnormal protein is not produced, which in the case of sickle cell disease is the abnormal Hemoglobin-S.

The potential antiaging methods involving genes fall into three broad categories:

- *gene therapy:* manipulating old and dysfunctional genes so that they act young and functional
- *gene editing:* removing genes that are the source of health problems
- *epigenetic editing:* turning on or off switches that control a specific gene without changing the gene

You may remember we attributed a lot of the progress in controlling aging to the Human Genome Project—an international research collaboration that set out to map and identify all of the genes in the human body. While the teams involved expected to find some 300,000 genes, they landed on about 22,500.

It cost $2.7 billion to sequence the genome at the time in the 1990s and early 2000s (it now costs a little more than $100 at Walmart to get a major part of your genome through Ancestry or 23andMe for you to map and ID your own genes). With the project, the research community had high hopes for gene therapy and gene editing as ways to treat disease and aging. (The breakthroughs experienced a major setback when a teen died during experimental trials with gene editing in 1999.)[10]

All of that work, development, and research revolved around a great hope and question: If we could identify the cells with gene perpetrators that commit biological crimes in our bodies, could we rehab them to be upstanding cellular citizens—or else perhaps sentence them to death?

If we could do either of those two things, we'd go a long way in being able to treat or prevent disease because we'd be able to change the function of our genes—turning something we initially believed to be predestined into something that was indeed editable or could even be rebooted back to its original state.

Groups from the Universities of California at Davis and San Diego, and at Harvard, MIT, and other institutions have achieved this with animals.[11] [12] This genetic reset has been achieved in mice in work by a company with researchers formerly from UC Davis and UC San Diego. These mice, which were bred to have advanced aging, had their genes reprogrammed. While it may be more difficult to visualize a young mouse, imagine rebooting your own 17-year-old dog to a puppy of age three, or your 60-year-old body to age 28—rebooting your operating system to be younger longer. That is what happened by simply (at least, it is simple in theory) restoring the controls of protein production to the state they were in for the mice in the studies.

Return the controls to where they were when you were young (to your original factory settings) and you make the mix of proteins young, and that makes you young. It took just changing the on/off position for four genes. Finding those genes was hard (a Japanese scientist, Shinya Yamanaka, was awarded the Nobel Prize for his work in finding them[13]), but turning the controls to just the right level of protein production from each was even harder: While turning on those genes made the mice young again, they soon developed cancer from the genes' uncontrolled growth. So the experiments in the laboratory took almost 14 years until the right amount and type of substances restored youth without increasing the risk of cancer. This is the concept of rebooting your epigenes (an epigenetic reboot, or a reset of the switches that determine which genes are on or not) to your original factory settings— and what makes this advance so promising.

In 2019, scientists reported that they had doubled the life span of roundworms by turning off one of the genes involved in aging.[14] In early life, the gene works by releasing a chemical that helps the organism grow and develop, but the theory is that, at a certain point, that chemical actually becomes counterproductive, contributing to age-related damage.[16] Turn off the gene after it stops being functionally helpful, and you reduce the damage and extend life. Added benefit: The worms also had healthier offspring. And while the worm life span only doubled from three weeks to six weeks, roundworms

Breakthrough Bonus

In late 2020, research showed that you could reverse eye aging by having cells repair themselves by tackling epigenetic changes that cause genes to express symptoms of aging.[15] Aging researcher David Sinclair and his team at Harvard, and others at Yale, the University of California at Los Angeles, and the University of New South Wales in Australia, used the eye to show that they could restore youthful DNA methylation and reverse vision loss in mice. The eye's retina and optic nerve regenerated themselves. But this means even more, much more: Reprogramming the methylation process in your cells can allow the cells to repair or replace themselves.

share 21 percent of the same DNA as humans and share many of the essential biological characteristics that are central to human biology, making this a very promising path for exploration. Now a group combining the resources of the MDI Biological Laboratory in Maine, the Buck Institute for Research on Aging in California, and Nanjing University in China have turned off two genes (IIS and TOR) and extended roundworms' life span by five (five!) times their normal age at death. If this happens with your longevity, age 400 is someday possible.[17]

The gene editing and the epigenetic on-and-off technologies are not perfect, but they are improving. About 10,000 diseases are caused by a single error in a single gene. In theory, we should be able to eliminate every one of them through gene editing. If you know the gene and the error, you can get rid of it.

Another vital point is the idea of self-engineering your genes through lifestyle decisions that flip the switches that control whether your genes are on or off. We are always changing the ways our genes function or are expressed. And we know now that behaviors—like exercise and eating—have influence over the way our genes work and which of those 1,500 genes are expressed (making their proteins) at any one time. In fact, you can engineer about 1,200 of them, making you the world's most prolific self-engineer (even if you flunked biology and chemistry).[18]

That's what we call turning genes "on," so they make proteins. This means that certain traits and functions aren't finite, but fluid—i.e., able to be influenced by outside factors. In particular, many lifestyle choices play a role in how and which genes are turned on, indicating that you can change your family history going forward. Hard as it is to believe, it's likely that you won't always be destined to be the product of your inherited genes.

It's now believed that aging—and specifically genes that age you—are turned on or off by a process called methylation and demethylation.[19] This process represses genes and keeps them from being activated or deactivated. Why is that important? Well, if aging is caused by expression of genes rather than damage to the genes themselves, we should be able to manipulate DNA affected by environmental factors and restore these controls of protein production to their youthful positions. This hypothesis is called the epigenetic model of aging.[20]

Think of your choices as the "settings" switches on your smartphone, tablet, or computer. There are literally thousands of things you could do to influence the performance of your tech—but you probably only choose or utilize a handful. The same applies to influencing the performance of your genes. But instead of tinkering with monitor brightness or Bluetooth settings, you are making lifestyle choices that switch your genes on and off to influence the way *your* machine works and ages. Of course, just as with your devices,

---

Breakthrough Bonus

Researchers are developing a new material to help get genetic editing tools directly into target cells—using a method that could be safer and cheaper than current modes of viral delivery. The new method uses what's called a "metal-organic framework" that's enhanced with a coating made of a green tea phytochemical.[21] This is important because it helps with delivery, the largest roadblock when it comes to capitalizing on the effectiveness of CRISPR editing of DNA.

the switches you control do not completely determine your DNA settings. Some—at least with present medical technology—are locked in DNA settings that are currently the focus of extensive genetic research.

Having the ability to methylate and demethylate switches that control genes gives you the ability to turn them off and on. Think of it like turning on or off gas burners on a stove or opening or closing an app on your phone or tablet; you could regulate your genes to express in a certain way. For instance, you could turn off genes that promote damaging inflammation or you could turn on genes that decrease inflammation.

In a way, this process is almost like the biological form of artificial intelligence: You can game your own genes to act in a way that you want, and change a less-than-optimal genetic history. And who wouldn't want that ability? It's not just to feel better (though that's a nice dividend). It's to extend your youthfulness by making your golden years truly golden: a longer time spent feeling, acting, and being young, no matter your calendar age.

This engineering occurs throughout a lifetime of daily decisions that you make. It occurs because of what you ate today—and the thousands of days before that. Those choices

Breakthrough Bonus

University of Virginia researchers have identified a gene that could go a long way in helping to prevent heart attacks.[22] While we've known for a long time that genetics plays a role in heart disease, these researchers have found a gene that has a protective effect on the heart—thus potentially opening up doors for developing new methods to help that gene be expressed to serve that function.

can make you healthy, which in itself will allow you to repair yourself when the time comes. Therefore, a lifetime of decisions—getting regular exercise or not, smoking or not, handling stress or not—can be the difference between whether you rocket up an incline, slog through it, or completely avoid it. (We cover the way you can turn your switches on and off in Part 4.)

And that will be a major component of what extends your youthful years and prevents chronic diseases so that you stay younger for longer. The ethical dilemmas that will arise from this revolutionary advance will make for both major scientific studies and sensational tabloid headlines. But self-engineering your genes does have exciting promise to help reduce and eliminate disease and dysfunction.

CHAPTER 6

IN YOUR DEFENSE

Could the advances in immunotherapy be the key to curing cancer and pandemics?

W hen a 58-year-old patient named Johnny was diagnosed with pancreatic cancer in Toronto in 2019, he was given six months to live. Essentially a death sentence. The only option to—perhaps—prolong his life was a tough chemotherapy regimen that would leave him in severe pain during his last days.

See, this pancreatic cancer—like so many forms of cancer—works by tricking a person's immune system so it stops fighting the cancer and allows those toxic cells to grow and kill healthy cells, eventually making systems and organs fail to the point where the person can't function any longer and dies.

Cancer engages in this high-stakes masquerade game perhaps from a mutation in a gene, disguising itself and infiltrating an area where it's not wanted—without being detected or asked to leave by a vigilant immune system whose job it is to get rid of unwanted invaders.

Johnny, without much hope for a cure, searched Clinical Trials.gov and entered a research trial in Houston (at the

MD Anderson Cancer Center) soon after his diagnosis. He had to argue to get into the trial, but he was a great advocate, as was his doc. As part of the experiment, researchers took two pints of his blood, then returned them to Johnny after they had harvested his immune cells from it.

The researchers then edited those cells (using the same CRISPR technology we discussed in the last chapter) and inserted into them a gene that made antibodies that could attack his specific pancreatic cancer.

It worked.

After a two-week period in which he felt severe flu-like symptoms (this was the immune system fighting the tumor), the tumor disappeared. Totally disappeared and hasn't come back. Johnny was cured.

This genetic manipulation of immune cells is one of the great frontiers in cancer treatment. It's a genetic chess game of sorts. As the cancer works by outsmarting the immune system, our move is to manipulate the immune system to outsmart the cancer. Checkmate?

We are only in early stages with some major successes. For example, metastatic malignant melanoma has gone from a disease with a one to 5 percent survival rate to a now 60-plus percent cure rate—and that's not just in research trials, but in real-life, clinical data. Not living with the tumor but cured!

This is where some of the most promising science lies, as immunotherapy advances have changed the way we think about treating cancer.[1] Rather than using a model of brute warfare like radiation and chemo to kill cancer—and with friendly fire killing some of the normal tissue near the cancer, too—we may in the future use therapies that teach our immune systems to protect healthy cells while destroying cancerous ones.

Why do cancer cells want to invade and destroy? For the same reason some people rob banks—to reap the benefits of living off other people's work. In this case, the perps take over your cells' energy in order to multiply and thrive.

So how can a rogue cell, a cancer cell, exist if you have a strong immune system? The cancer cell plays a game of identity theft by sending out a signal that it's one of your good, healthy cells, so that the immune system does not attack it.

Your immune system has many levels of defense. Some of your immune cells fight. Some cells in your immune army die in the fight, and some work on the intelligence aspect of defense, taking inventory of the recent battle so that they can better identify potential threats in the future. And some of your immune system works to carry away debris from the fight, aided by proteins called resolvins.[2]

If all goes well in a typical defense scenario, the invader comes in, the invader is identified, the fight happens, the

Breakthrough Bonus

Researchers at University College London have moved one step closer to being able to build a human thymus—a key organ in the immune system. If you have a dysfunctional thymus you can't fight off disease and infection as well; if a transplanted thymus—with full function—were available, it could help stave off a variety of diseases. The researchers have rebuilt a thymus using stem cells.[3]

immune system wins, and the debris is shuttled away from the site and out of the body via your lymph system. Your immune system then takes a break (it really is still rooting out rogue cancer cells, which are developing all the time) and prepares for the next alarm. This is what happens in the case of a common cold, for example; the symptoms (coughing, sneezing, etc.) are not the cold; they are the result of the immune fight. Those symptoms demonstrate that your body is working to expel the invader.

But when some cancer cells get smart and send out that signal to your immune system that they are really normal cells, the signal goes to what is termed a checkpoint ("immune system, check yourself because I am really an OK cell"). Cancer cells skirt the security system—and left unchecked, they duplicate and grow.

Your immune system doesn't know to recognize those cancer cells as threats. And the cancer—feeding off friendly cells—grows and grows (and often spreads) until it starts destroying your body's cells and organs.

So much of cancer treatment thus far has centered on the direct destruction of cancer cells through surgery, radiation, and chemotherapy (which can destroy healthy cells in the process). But the most promising advances in cancer research and treatment today center on immunotherapy—that is, empowering and activating the body's own immune system to identify and attack the cancer cells.

That, at least at this point and in the foreseeable future, would seem to be the gold standard: Have your immune system attack cancer cells the way it attacks the common cold or a seasonal flu. A short fight with no long-term negative effects. One of the newer advances researchers are now testing is what was used in Johnny's successful battle with pancreatic cancer: insertion of a gene into lymphocytes that enhances their anti-tumor and cell-killing effectiveness—that means insertion of a gene that helps your immune system find and kill tumor cells better.

Immunotherapy works by stimulating the body's immune system to better fight cancer cells and by boosting parts of the immune system to prevent the formation of cancer (working like a vaccine).

For cancer treatment, the immunotherapy techniques are generally classified into five buckets:

- *general immune-boosting behaviors* (which can theoretically help your system better fight cancer), like getting enough sleep and eating sufficient micronutrients[4][5][6]
- *man-made antibodies* (antibodies designed to attack specific cells)
- *vaccines* (put into the body to trigger an immune response; these would help prevent certain cancers)
- *checkpoint inhibitors* (which allow the immune system to not be tricked by cancer cells, so it can better recognize and fight them)
- *insertion of genes into immune cells* to help them target and kill cancer cells more effectively (as was the case with Johnny)

While these approaches are in various stages of development and are even being used in some cancer treatments, we find the checkpoint and gene insertion approaches to be two of the most fascinating—especially with their implications for how the immune system works.

In the 1970s, a grad student named Jim Allison posed a central question: There must be a reason the immune system doesn't attack cancer, and that must be that some cancer cells send out a signal that essentially deactivates the immune system. How?

Allison was singing the "immunotherapy blues" (extra credit: Do a Google search to see Jim's *Rolling Stone*–style magazine cover in 2001), because one-year effective rates of immunotherapy in many trials were zero—no different from chemotherapy alone. And he wondered, why is it working in animals and not humans?

But he persisted and insisted on a three-year head-to-head trial of immunotherapy with chemotherapy versus chemotherapy alone. After three years, the effectiveness of immunotherapy and chemo was far higher than the effects of chemo alone because of the way the immune system functioned to fight the cancer.[7]

Allison, who went on to win the 2018 Nobel Prize in Physiology or Medicine (and became chair of immunotherapy at MD Anderson), is credited with developing a way to attack cancer not by treating the disease, but by treating the immune system. The key insight was to block the protein in cancer cells that slams the brakes on immune cells called T cells. That allows T cells to get past the "checkpoint" and attack cancer. Allison's work led to the development of the first checkpoint inhibitor drugs (the first of which was used for metastatic malignant melanoma). His band is now known as the Checkpoints.

Others have added substantially to this "checkpoint work" to make important contributions to cancer-free survival, notably the group at Dana-Farber Cancer Institute that discovered the second type of checkpoint inhibitors, PDL-1 checkpoint inhibitors.[8] While the current checkpoint inhibitors are effective at helping treat solid-tissue tumors that are rapidly dividing (like metastatic malignant melanoma), the future focuses are on other types of tumors, like blood-borne, slowly developing chronic lymphocytic leukemias.

The point: Immunotherapy is like many things in health. You need some time (three years, in this case) to show the benefit, and you shouldn't always give up if initial results (multiple one-year trials in this case) aren't promising.

Immunotherapy techniques are a far better answer to cancer than some of the prior models because they don't kill healthy cells. Instead, they look to improve the function of the defense systems, so that they can do the job they are intended to do: destroy what does not belong without hurting anything else in the process. We expect many cancers will have better cure rates by 2030 as researchers develop ways for your immune system to attack more effectively.

VIRUSES AND VACCINES

When it comes to your health and longevity, there's a good chance that your immune system is at the top of your mind. Certainly, the COVID-19 pandemic that began in 2020 made us think about how we can survive and fight off attacks from viral invaders.[9]

Your body—smart little sucker that it is—is born with an excellent defense strategy. It protects what is most valuable in order to thrive for the future: itself. During the first year of the COVID-19 pandemic, more than 80 percent of those under age 70 in the United States who needed ICU care (and more than 90 percent of those who died) had one of six largely preventable co-morbid conditions: obesity, less than perfectly treated hypertension or cardiovascular disease, type 2 diabetes, immune dysfunction, or smoking- (or vaping-) induced lung disease.[10]

All of these conditions degrade your defenses. If you live in a developed country, you can make simple choices (like getting regular sleep or making specific nutritional choices or managing stress, or engaging in physical activity) that improve your immune defenses against SARS-CoV-2—and all other invaders or miscreant cells.[5] That said, much has been discussed about vaccines and viruses—how to slow the spread of a massive threat to individuals and societal longevity. Some important questions about the subject:

How does COVID-19 invade?

With SARS-CoV-2, the virus attacks a specific type of cell in your nasal passages (ciliary cells), as well as in your lungs (pneumocyte-2s).[11] The latter produce a chemical that keeps the air sacs in your lungs open so they can help provide you with oxygen. In the coronavirus fight, sometimes the immune system goes into hyperdrive, creating an inflammation that breaks off plaques in your arteries and can even cause other friendly fire like pneumonia, which further destroys oxygenating ability—a double whammy on your oxygen intake. If your immune system is strong and rested (yes, sleep, meditation, exercise, and food choices are important to the capability of your system), you win.

If all goes well, your immune system takes a break and prepares for the next alarm. COVID-19 is deadly because it preys on people with low immunity (and, by duplicating in those cilia in your outer nose, spreads more easily than the prior SARS virus, which only duplicates in the lung cells and not in the more available nasal ciliary cells). It also creates another distinct problem—some people (long haulers, as they're called) make antibodies to the virus that destroy or attack their own tissues. That means the virus can cause disease long after it is gone. We need a vaccine that doesn't cause you to produce an immune response that causes an attack on other parts of your body. Scientists seem to have found many vaccines that cause you to produce antibodies that stop coronavirus with very rare side effects (less than 1 in 100,000 even in the most vulnerable groups) of attacking healthy tissues.

How does a vaccine work?

Unlike antibiotics, which work to attack an existing invader, vaccines upgrade and boost your immune system.[12] They teach your body about certain antigens so your body develops antibodies and other immune-boosting processes—ones that can potentially ID threats and invaders, as well as ones that attack them. In essence, these immune cells form a massive identification system to build the troops (both other immune cells and antibodies) designed to fight specific threats.

Specifically, it's the B cells that produce antibodies to fight off invaders and call upon T cells to help fight, and it's the B cells that are stimulated by vaccines. If the vaccine works wonders, these B cells turn into a few plasma cells that lie in wait in your bone marrow for the viral or bacterial invader. When they are triggered, they do not let the virus or bacteria enter a cell to take over its (your cellular) reproductive machinery.

HIV and some other viruses have escaped successful vaccine development due to their ability to mutate or build a protective coat, which decreases the ability of your B cells to intervene.[13]

In SARS-CoV-2, antibodies against the non-attaching portions of the virus don't stop the virus from entering your cells and multiplying; you need specific antibodies (called neutralizing antibodies) that block the attachment to the cell so the virus can't get into it to replicate.

What about antiviral medication?

These medications work by attacking non-attachment points of the virus (for HIV, most work inside your cells to attack the HIV virus and stop its spread after the virus particles have replicated). However, the preferred route is to stop the virus from getting inside your cells in the first place.

Why does it take so long to produce a vaccine?

Typically, vaccines have taken 10 to 20 years to produce (at least they did before the search for a COVID-19 vaccine).[14] The goals of vaccine development are, first of all, safety and, second, to induce the kind of immune response that is necessary to prevent infection and disease due to the specific pathogen; distinct pathogens can require different mechanisms to provide protective immunity. Especially in a pandemic, rapid, large-scale production is absolutely essential. We need billions of doses of any COVID-19 vaccine. And we need to be able to economically deliver them on a global scale.

Another goal, especially in the case of COVID-19, is a vaccine that blocks the infection where the virus enters the body and the cell. Since we know that SARS-CoV-2 ordinarily enters through the respiratory tract—the mouth or nose—we want immunity that operates right there at the portal of entry and not just in the bloodstream. And we want to develop a vaccine that generates at least a year of immunological memory. Ideally, vaccines will induce immune responses that recognize viral targets that can't mutate to escape; flu viruses change their frequency often and mutate so our immunity doesn't last for long, which is why we have to get a new shot yearly (though there is now in testing a long-lasting flu vaccine that induces antibodies that attack a non-mutating part of the virus).[15] Finally, vaccines need to be stable enough for worldwide distribution—a vaccine that requires freezing or even refrigeration is not going to reach everyone—which is why many different vaccines have been developed for SARS-CoV-2.

In addition, a new vaccine has to work in the real world (not just trials) with large, diverse populations, including (especially) minorities, those with comorbidities, and the elderly. All of these factors and steps can be rushed only to a limited extent.

Efficacy studies follow safety studies—they usually take one to two years to complete, and determine if the vaccine offers protection. They can be done in very large populations at risk—some are vaccinated and others are given a placebo vaccination and then the rates of infection in the two groups are compared. That's expensive, and it can be complicated by fluctuations in the frequency of the disease in question. For example, if a flu vaccine trial was started after the peak of flu season, the rate of infection in both groups might be too low to find a difference in infection rates.

The alternative is a human challenge study, but exposing people to a deadly virus might not get a lot of sane volunteers.[16] In the challenge, some people are vaccinated, some are not, and all are then challenged with the real SARS-CoV-2 virus. Challenge studies are generally done with viruses for which there's a readily available curative therapy—a bug that causes diarrhea, for example. You watch for evidence that a person develops diarrhea and treat them immediately with therapies that prevent complications and that kill the bug. We haven't had that advantage in the case of the new coronavirus, since during vaccine development we didn't have a highly effective treatment.[17] [18]

What is the future of pandemics?

The antivirals and new vaccine platforms developed during COVID-19 are what give us hope that we can prevent pandemics from killing one to 10 percent of the population, as they did in the distant past. Safety testing for coronavirus vaccines is more detailed because one of the initial candidates in the preparation of vaccines for the original SARS caused a hyper-immune reaction that put a very few (but a few) vaccine recipients at risk of serious complications—so the testing was improved. That improved, safer process, as well as more development of antiviral medications, will make the dangers of a new pandemic lower, but clearly not zero. The fact that the new SARS-CoV-2 vaccines may be available for more than three billion people (four to six billion doses) in less than two years shows incredible progress in preventing a pandemic from shortening longevity.[19]

CHAPTER 7

THE FUTURE OF YOUR ENERGY

How your body's power sources can extend your prime time

n a world where on-off switches are ubiquitous, it's easy to see why such a switch could be so appealing biologically speaking. Just as you saw with the epigenetic switches, turning pathways on and off can help your body.

Turn on what you want. Turn off what you don't.

In August 2020, an international research team reported that they had discovered how to activate something called brown fat. No, brown fat isn't some kind of effect that comes from wolfing down too much chocolate ice cream. It's actually one of the keys to metabolism, controlling obesity and diabetes, and perhaps longevity. The results of the collaboration between the Centre de recherche du Centre hospitalier universitaire de Sherbrooke (CRCHUS) in Québec and the Novo Nordisk Foundation Center for Basic Metabolic Research (CBMR) at the University of Copenhagen were published in the journal *Cell Metabolism*.[1]

Brown fat burns energy and generates heat—a process called thermogenesis—after being activated by cold temperatures or chemical signals. Humans have small deposits of brown fat, and scientists have long hypothesized that finding alternative ways to pharmacologically activate that fat or turn white fat into brown fat could help improve metabolism.

In this chapter, we'll look not only at the role of this fat (a form of energy storage), but also at the energy factories that really power your body at the cellular level (mitochondria). These energy systems serve as a key piece of the puzzle when it comes to life-extending advances.

Reframing Fat

We are living in an unprecedented era of obesity, particularly in the U.S., and the negative impacts of excess fat are well known. In 1960, only 11 percent of adult males were obese or extremely obese. Today, it is 43 percent.[2] Among adult females it rose from 17 percent to 54 percent. In the U.S. today, 50 percent of non-Hispanic adult blacks are obese or extremely obese, as are 45 percent of Hispanic blacks, 42 percent of non-Hispanic whites, and 18 percent of Asians. And among children ages two through 19, the obesity rate is 19 percent.

When you eat too much, extra glucose or calories of almost any kind turn into triglycerides, which turn into fat. Extra fat in your belly makes you more insulin-resistant and at greater risk for developing diabetes, and increases inflammation and rupture of atherosclerotic plaques in you.[3] When atherosclerotic plaques rupture, the calcified plaque can travel downstream, leading to clogged arteries. And on the newly raw plaque surface, platelets gather to smooth the ruptured area, attracting a lattice network of clotting factors and red blood cells—resulting in a partially or totally obstructed artery. In these ways, fat has been shown to contribute to a malfunctioning of circulatory circuitry, increasing the possibility of clogged arteries, strokes, and many other forms of heart and brain problems. The inflammation visceral or belly fat causes also exacerbates osteoarthritis, depression, and stress; causes fatigue from a variety of disorders from sleep apnea to dementia; and is a major cause of six cancers, including breast and colon. So unless you're a sumo champ or an offensive lineman (and even then it can get you!), it's safe to assume that fat in your viscera (belly) is a bad thing. Remember that fat is a way that we store energy in case we need it. The problem is that our storage tanks in 2021 as opposed to those we had prior to 1950 are stretched beyond reason.

But not all fat is created equal. The fat most people picture is known as white fat, since it looks white or white-yellow when you see it under the skin. But you're also born with brown fat (which, unsurprisingly, looks brown).[4]

Brown fat—found in the neck and shoulders of newborns—is metabolically efficient, in that it burns lots of calories, which serves the purpose of keeping you warm (important for newborns). We lose our brown fat as we age. By age six, you have less than 5 percent of the brown fat you were born with; the fat we gain over time is almost all white fat. White fat is metabolically inefficient, meaning it's relatively inactive—it doesn't use much energy, and in addition it is hard to burn off, accumulates, and causes those other health problems like inflammation we refer to above.

So what does this have to do with youthfulness?

Well, researchers at a company near UC Davis and

separately at the University of Copenhagen have taken white fat in test tubes, regressed it to a more pluripotent fat, flipped a few epigenetic switches, and—*voilà!*—turned it into brown fat. They then injected the brown fat into fat sheep. What happened? As hoped, the sheep with more brown fat got thin and lost their metabolic syndrome and diabetes.

One roadblock to using brown fat is that all the good stuff that brown fat does has to be programmed into the previously white fat, but that has proved doable. A group in Delaware has done this white-fat-to-brown-fat transformation by activating dormant brown fat in a few women in a small way with an already approved medication. That could lead to research to develop a related but newer medication; it could also lead to a set of stem cell and exosome transplants that can transform more of your white fat to much more metabolically active brown fat to help get rid of unwanted fat and pounds to a greater degree in a reliable way. Most older people don't have significant amounts of brown fat. So you need to do more than just activate the brown fat you have—you need more brown fat.

But what if, as they did at that company near UC Davis and at the University of Copenhagen, scientists could do this in a person rather than just in a test tube—that is, what if a person's white fat could be turned into brown fat, through what is called induced tissue regeneration—using reprogramming to transform one cell type to pluripotent cells (see Chapter 3), and then specific genes could be turned on to make those cells function like brown fat cells? And what if those newly made brown fat cells could then get injected back into the person?

This process requires two distinct and really important

discoveries. As we noted earlier, induced pluripotent stem cells from adult cells hold great promise. Dr. Shinya Yamanaka in Japan reverted adult cells to their original embryonic state (at which point they could turn into many different cells such as brown fat, or white fat, or heart or brain or kidney, etc.). Dr. Yamanaka did this reversion by turning on four genes (now called the Yamanaka factors), which he accomplished by activating four embryonic switches.[5]

So, after reverting adult white fat cells into pluripotent cells, the research group then made a few more epigenetic switches to make brown fat cells. They then grew the brown fat cells in culture and made them non-immunogenic by turning on another switch (the gene that controls the HLA-G genome) that changed the expression of proteins on the cells' surface.[6] That made it possible to inject the brown fat back into fat sheep without the sheep rejecting it.

The timetable for this game-changing ability to turn white fat to brown fat is predicted to be less than five years away after human studies start. The brown fat will likely make you much thinner; reduce your risk of diabetes, heart disease, cancer, osteoarthritis, and dementia; and maybe make eating a lot of ice cream OK again. That's a major wow moment: Fatter folks could become thin with this change alone.

Why is this important? Since 1974, one of the major causes of shortened life spans and of both disease itself and the uptick in chronic illnesses like osteoarthritis, type 2 diabetes, and many cancers is that increasing level of white fat (our genes haven't changed since 1974—but our choices, which influence which of our genes are activated, have, resulting in enormous medical costs). Many of the symptoms of aging, even fatigue and a lack of energy, are derived from the biological destruction and inflammation that comes from excess white fat. The accumulation of white fat in society has resulted in a life expectancy that is shorter than it would be. And while medical treatments have mitigated much of the disease and life expectancy change caused by white fat, we continue as a society (and often individually) to accumulate excess white fat. Much of that increase comes from eating the five food felons, including foods that have saturated fats and foods that produce an increase in blood sugar levels too quickly (like cupcakes). The five felons are added sugar, syrups, simple or non-100 percent whole grains, foods with saturated fat (due to the amino acids they have), and trans fats. Replace white fat with brown fat and you've most likely greatly reduced the risks of all inflammatory diseases like osteoarthritis, diabetes, heart disease, stroke, and brain dysfunction and have increased energy levels. That is, you become operationally younger. This change alone would make your Reboot age as much as 20 years younger than your RealAge at age 75. Bring it on!

Energy of Your Cells: Mitochondria

If the last time you heard the word "mitochondria" was in biology class or when Uncle Lenny guessed wrong while watching *Jeopardy!*, you may need a quick refresher course.

Mitochondria are small contained units within your cells that function as your body's power plants.[7] When all is said and done, it's the mitochondria that are responsible for giving you the energy to make your body run. Since everything that happens in your body requires energy—heart beating, stomach digesting, brain thinking, muscles moving—you need a constant supply of juice, which comes in the form of the chemical

ATP. The mitochondria in each cell provide that juice by processing the glucose and fat from the food you eat. Those mitochondria convert glucose and fat into ATP, which is the jolt that is sent to your organs and systems to make everything run.

Now, with just about everything that happens in your body, there are some trade-offs that occur during everyday functioning. Making energy creates waste, like exhaust from a car. That's the byproduct of running the engine.

Your cells work the same way, but this biological exhaust comes in the form of what are called free radicals, which are chemicals that can damage your cells. The DNA in your mitochondria produces the proteins that help make energy. What governs whether that DNA in your mitochondria is producing proteins efficiently is the damage over the years from those free radicals. What governs whether that protein factory is on or off is the damage or changes in DNA that turn your DNA factory on or off. These are the epigenetic DNA switches, which also are damaged by free radicals. So there are two sets of potential damage to make it less likely you'll have the energy to keep up with your grandkids.

Your body tries to remove free radicals via antioxidants, which try to bind the free radicals up (as if they were in handcuffs) and haul them out of your cells and then out of your body. That's one of the reasons blueberries and exercise are so good for you—they are two very powerful ways to increase your in-cell antioxidants. Regularly drinking black coffee is another.[8] There are only three in-cell antioxidants, and most food antioxidants do not increase them. Fortunately, blueberries, regular black coffee, N-acetyl cysteine, a few other supplements, and physical activity have been proven to do so. These allow you to genetically self-engineer, and you don't even need the help of MIT or Cal-Tech.

So, the price you pay for having a body that works is some waste product. It's not unlike other aspects of life; it's the price of biological business. All things being equal, the system runs pretty well. Power plant on, energy to organs, waste products produced, waste products bound by the in-cell antioxidants and shoveled off.

But, like airports in a thunderstorm, or power plants or transmission lines in a deep freeze, not everything always runs smoothly.

Problems occur when you have too much glucose or fat (i.e., you eat too many calories—Thanksgiving? Super Bowl Sunday? Every day?). Too much glucose and fat overwhelm the body's ability to have in-cell antioxidants clear all the free radicals—so the free radicals are, well, free to do damage to your DNA. You can probably predict the effect: When the power generator or the switches that control that generator are damaged, you create less energy, and your systems slow down, don't work as well, and eventually lose their function. Over time, when your mitochondria are fried, you run out of energy. That's when you become frail and can't function as well as you once did.

Currently, scientists in Lausanne; Ottawa; Zurich; Mumbai; Cambridge, Massachusetts; Baltimore; and São Paulo are looking at how to restore and reboot your mitochondria via that same process used to transform white fat into brown fat: induced tissue regeneration.[9][10] The current cell with its damaged mitochondria is regressed to a cell of the type you had at birth. That way those cells and mitochondria can function as if they're new and youthful power plants, providing a strong source of energy and prolonging the time before they fail or die off. Just imagine if that could be done to all your cells outside of your brain. You could have the energy you had when you were a teenager but keep all your intelligence. And, yes, live younger longer. That is the promise of induced tissue regeneration of your mitochondria.

Some research has determined that the malfunctioning of mitochondria is part of aging and of specific diseases often triggered by fever. Keeping mitochondria healthy (less sugar, less saturated fat, smaller meals, and less white fat promoting inflammation) slows down this aging process as we know it. And you end up with more energy every day. If your cells—via your power source—can become or stay much younger-acting, then your organs and systems will function much more youthfully, decreasing the chances of developing disease.

Advancements in mitochondria restoration and rebooting show that we can alter our biology to make our cells young acting, even if they're old by the standards of calendar age— sometimes by replacing nutrients in the mitochondria that have declined with aging, like NAD (see page 238 for more explication of the role of NAD and its decline with aging).[11] Rebooting makes animals act with the energy of their much younger selves. In one experiment scientists in Switzerland injected a precursor form of NAD called NR into mice with genetic Alzheimer's and reversed the mental dysfunction.[12]

Though no such benefit has been published for human cognitive dysfunction (studies are in progress), we do know that people with cognitive dysfunction have decreased levels of NAD, and that a precursor to NAD is safe for humans to take as a supplement in short-term studies (see page 238). That is why so many researchers in the aging field now take this supplement. Restoring mitochondrial health, the cellular foundation for all of our biological functions, in older people is a frontier that can have huge implications in the quality of how your body operates.

CHAPTER 8

BIONIC BODIES

How new technology may be able to save or replace bad body parts

You already have a good idea of how a heart attack happens: Plaque builds up in the walls of your arteries (as a result of unhealthy lifestyle choices and/or because of genetics). The plaque acts like a roadblock as it narrows your arteries and causes your blood to change direction and lanes. In its final stage it narrows the arteries so much that not enough blood can travel to and from your heart. And when blood can't flow, oxygen is cut off, and that's when a heart attack or stroke happens.

Of course, we now have a number of ways to treat heart attacks—we can clear or reroute the arteries through a variety of surgical interventions (stents, bypasses). But these methods come with a heavy cost: catheterization, open-heart surgery, extensive rehab, a compromised circulatory system.

Today, researchers are working on new, ideally more effective and less intrusive ways to destroy plaque before it clogs and creates obstructions that can cause permanent damage.

Though it sounds like it could be a video game, the idea is that you could send MRI-guided nanorobots into the blood vessels that could grab the plaque, bust it into little pieces, and have it excreted by the body, as well as repair the damaged blood vessels. (*Who you gonna call? PLAQUE BUSTERS!*) The challenge researchers are facing is to break up the plaque so it doesn't travel downstream to cause injury somewhere else.[1]

The use of nanobots is being tested in small animals in a lab near Palo Alto, California. Rats and rabbits bred to develop atherosclerosis are exposed to stresses that promote plaque—making a rat swim for hours to stay alive is like making you swim for days to stay alive. That activity is stressful enough to promote the rapid development of atherosclerotic plaques in arteries.

Then scientists anesthetize the animals, put them in MRI machines, locate their plaque, send in a bot, and give the bot the tools to gobble the plaque.

The plaque disappears without the need for surgery.

We don't know if those rats or rabbits feel better afterward, but for humans, the potential with this kind of treatment is that you could possibly avoid the ICU and lots of rehab that is required after having open-heart surgery to bypass an artery.

Some more examples of new tech:

Organ or tissue regeneration: A Harvard professor is working on a technique that would allow the ACL (a ligament in the knee) to heal on its own, rather than via replacement with a tendon from another person or animal, or from another part of your body.

This technique involves inserting an hourglass-shaped sponge filled with the patient's blood and growth factors and reactivated stem cells to act as a bridge between the two torn pieces.[2] The bridge parts grow and reconnect the tear, so you don't have to go through an intrusive repair using other soft tissue. The implications here go beyond simply improving sports performance; the procedure might also help reduce the incidence of later-life arthritis that often follows current ACL repairs in athletes (as well as in us non-athletes).

Artificial organs: We may be inching closer to what might be considered the gold standard of longevity advances: a genetically regenerated heart or artificial heart. Researchers at the Cleveland Clinic believe that if they had unlimited dollars, they could be less than three years away from growing a heart and inserting it into humans.

We're already sort of seeing this happen with the work on 3D printing of organs—producing mechanisms and materials that can function like tissue (even lung-like tissues, which develop COVID-19 like real lungs do and so can be used to study potential treatments and antivirals).[3] An Australian company recently developed a robotic device that prints a person's own skin cells, which could be used to repair skin damage from wounds or burns.[4]

Just imagine you could have a computer code for all your body parts stored in the cloud—and that you could use that information to create 3D-printed versions that could be swapped in as necessary. Cut that bone cancer out and replace the bone in question with a new version of equal shape, size, and strength and with the same connections to ligaments, joints, and other bones. That could be possible within 10 years.

Protein manipulation: What if you could engineer an organ or body part to regrow, or could manipulate the way the body works normally? In Korea, for example, researchers are testing antiaging drugs that alter the activity of proteins in round-worm cells; they work by telling the body to convert sugar into energy when cellular energy is running low (the worms got a life span boost with this technology).[5]

Fix-it tools: A good way to think about how technological advances can work in the longevity ecosystem is to consider how far we've come in the area of heart valves, which wear out over time. About 10 percent of people 85 to 95 years of age (and more for people older) will have to have valves repaired or replaced, while 25 percent of people over 65 already have some kind of change in the function of the valves. The procedure to replace valves used to involve open-heart surgery, which, because it required stopping the heart and using a pump to circulate your blood, carried grave risk. Six months after open heart-valve surgery, 17 percent of patients had a decline in mental function.[6]

Today, minimally invasive surgery can replace a valve by feeding it into the heart through a blood vessel. Granted, it's still *heart* surgery, so it's still serious, but this common procedure allows a much faster recovery period.[7] We'll need to

Breakthrough Bonus

Researchers in Zurich have developed what's called "microvehicles" that can move though blood vessels to deliver medications.[8] They are robots so tiny (.25 millimeter) that they can travel through our bodies via our circulatory system. This development could change medicine significantly—as microvehicles could be used to treat aneurysms or even help perform certain surgical procedures.

replace many more valves if people live 20 to 30 years longer, so it's good news that the science of replacement seems to be getting ahead of our aging.

The next level of advancement in valve maintenance revolves around not repair nor replacement, but delaying the wear and tear that happens when the valves flap against each other up to 100 times a minute. Technology has played a major role in replace-or-repair solutions, but what if we got better at delaying the problem from even happening?

High-tech toys: Artificial intelligence, virtual reality, updated technology, improved data collection, and the like will also be game-changers in how we think about our health—and what we can do. We already have apps that can connect us to doctors for immediate consultations—telemedicine, essential during the COVID-19 shutdown. These apps allow remote medical care, which was previously impossible. But what happens when next-gen technology takes hold? Better collection of data could lead to better development of drugs. Wearable technology could not just track what you've done but predict your future. Artificial intelligence could predict that valve wearing out before it causes you any problem. More accessible diagnostics could mean delaying problems down the road.

A Yale genetics researcher has developed a handheld ultrasound device.[9] While it doesn't quite have as high definition as the $100,000 ultrasound machine, the $2,000 device could make scanning as easy and common for wellness visits as listening to your heart and neck has been for doctors. Such scanning should help docs know on whom to push prevention or who to motivate to make healthier choices.

We will see explosive growth in all corners of the tech industry. A recent report from CNBC said that the "delaying death" market is expected to grow to $600 billion with emphases on such things as big data, artificial intelligence, gene editing, food engineering, and cure-diseases medications (called "moonshot medicine").[10] And while the initial costs of these "delaying death" breakthroughs will be high, as with past innovations, their real cost will fall rapidly over time. What was once science fiction becomes an expensive reality, then ultimately an easily affordable, widespread practice. (The real moonshot by the Global Wellness Institute is "Eliminating Preventable Disease," which we cover in Part 4.)

So while many of our advances revolve around the cellular or genetic processes of aging, we will also see continuous and exponential physical, mechanical, and technological advances—changes that will extend our healthy life span, improve the quality of all life from middle age onward, and most likely at least double our prime years.

We may not end up with one magic pill or one-stop shop for living younger longer, but all of these advances combined will contribute to a 360-degree approach to longevity. You never know what new technology or which new development will be the one that will save or change your life—and help you be younger today and down the road.

PART 3

THE WEALTH AND HEALTH EFFECTS

What increased longevity will do for society, for your body, and for your life

What does all of this mean? How will these technological medical changes influence your body, as well as all of the factors that go along with such sweeping health changes, like societal and personal economics, your career, and more?

These next chapters will look at the implications of the Great Age Reboot, and how society will likely adjust to become more vibrant, productive, and prosperous.

Are there challenges with such massive changes? Of course. And it's difficult to see how everything will sync together—your life, government regulations, an entire medical community, and global economics. But this new way of life can work. And we predict that life, longevity, our bodies, and our society will look a heck of a lot different in the decades to come because of it.

| CHAPTER 9 |

BANKING ON THE GREAT AGE REBOOT

How will we pay for longer and younger lives?

B esides health, the second thing that scares the digested beans out of us about longevity? Running out of money.[1] And that circumstance has three aspects:

- Will we as individuals have saved enough and invested it wisely enough to last if we live decades longer than we imagined when we were younger?
- With the current emphasis on federal debt financing, will the inflation rate skyrocket and render our savings too small to support our longevity?
- Will governments have enough money to continue to pay for pensions (Social Security) and medical care of the elderly?

There's good reason for these concerns. The numbers, as they currently stand, are indeed worrisome. Although those over

50 are better prepared for retirement than any previous generation, few have saved enough to handle the medical expenses and long-term care costs associated with getting older. And the prospect of living longer without *enough* money sounds about as appealing as bark-flavored toothpaste. The coronavirus has shown what can happen if society or individuals do not have plans in place and sufficient savings when they are needed.

So how can you prepare for extended decades? And how can society prepare to handle the changes in infrastructure that will occur as millions and millions more people live longer?

We think the prospects are bright financially. In this chapter, we'll walk you through the societal and personal economics of the Great Age Reboot. And when you see the numbers, you'll understand how it all can come together—and what you can do to make this monumental shift work for you.

Today, working to age 65 is the norm (and most 65-year-olds are highly functioning and performing, we might add!). Nevertheless, it's difficult for us to imagine 80- or 90-year-olds as a major part of the workforce, since life expectancy now is 78 to 81. But what if that 90 or 100 becomes the new 40 or 55? At the very least, you can probably picture more and more 75-year-olds being vibrant parts of the workforce, because it is happening every day.

When you reboot your body, you can also extend your economic potential, your prime years. And when that happens, you can feel the shift—from fear to opportunity: the opportunity to live longer, healthier, *and* financially secure. Just as important, extending your prime years has a great overall effect on society. So taking care of yourself is not just an act of self-preservation; it can be viewed as an altruistic one as well. A better you means a better us. Let's examine how.

Societal Economics

How will we know what happens to the amount of money available for aging populations, Social Security, and medical care without first understanding what happens to the number of people who are contributing to the economy? To understand the economic implications of the reboot, we first have to dive into population projections.

While the average U.S. life span has declined over four of the last five years due to the opioid and pandemic crises and the influx of chronic disease due to obesity, the longevity progression continues for non-opioid users and non-obese people.[2] The routine increases in longevity that result from better illness treatments—such as statins to prevent heart disease and immunotherapy for cancer—as well as the exponential ones resulting from the biotech revolution and previously unimaginable medical advances, will be what drives increased life expectancy over the long term. In turn, that will mean faster-than-expected population growth, even if birth rates decline.

U.S. Census Bureau actuaries project that in 2050, the U.S. population will be about 55.5 million more than it is today, reaching a level of about 390 million.[3] Others think it will be less due to the changes in fertility. They argue that since life expectancy is declining in developed countries, populations will plunge. While that has happened in prior pandemics (and we have three in the United States—opioid, obesity, and SARS-CoV-2), as we noted in Chapter 1, life expectancy has rebounded fast in the past. When we adjust these estimates to reflect longer, rebooted life expectancies, we think this number will not be 55.5 million as predicted by the Census actuaries but closer to 117.5 million, with a potential to reach 451 million people (again we will refer to our projections as GARP, or Great Age Reboot Projections). This growth is due to a decrease in deaths rather than an increase in births.

Our numbers are based on similar birth and immigration rates as the Census Bureau estimates, but with a substantially decreased death rate for those 50 to 90-plus due to the medical progress and improvements in treating chronic disease.

In other words, even if birth rates decline (but total births increase slightly due to more people in the baby-producing ages) and immigration stabilizes over the next 30 years, we believe that greater longevity will add 62 million more people to the population than predicted by Census Bureau projections, bringing the total additions closer to 117.5 million more people. And for the most part, this cohort will be living robust and highly productive lives until their final five to 15 years (as is the case today). That is, they may be 70, 80, 90, or 100 years old chronologically, but they will have the energy and physical capacity we associate with being 15 to 35 (or more) years younger. Yes, if 60 is the new 40, now 95 or 100 will be the new 45 by 2050.

The chart shows how we estimate the U.S. population will break down by age by 2050. (For a more detailed look at population projections, see the chart on page 28.)

U.S. POPULATION CHANGE BY AGE

Age	2020 Population (millions)	2050 Reboot (GARP) Population (millions)	2050 U.S. Census Bureau Population (millions)
0–9	40.7	43.3	43.3
10–19	42.4	43.9	43.9
20–29	45.4	47.3	47.3
30–39	44.7	49.7	48.7
40–49	40.7	50.5	49.0
50–59	42.7	50.8	48.4
60–69	39.4	46.1	43.1
70–79	25.0	37.6	33.3
80–89	10.3	35.0	23.6
90–99	2.3	29.1	7.9
100–109	0.0	13.0	0.4
110–119	0.0	4.1	0.0
120+	0.0	0.5	0.0
Totals	**333.6**	**451.0**	**388.9**

We estimate that by 2050, more than 10 percent of the U.S. population will be 90 years or older—chronologically—and 18 percent will be over age 80. By way of comparison, in 1960 only 9.2 percent of the population was over 64 years old. But instead of hurting the economy and the government's ability to afford their Social Security and Medicare, these *yolds* (young olds) will increase society's resources to pay for these benefits. More people will be spending more time in what are effectively their prime years, earning more and paying taxes and contributing to Social Security, etc. The charts above and below show not just the dramatic increase in numbers, but the dramatic increase in the number of people on the older end of the spectrum. People 19 and younger made up 25 percent of the U.S. population in 2020. In 2050, this group will make up 19 percent of the population, a 24 percent decrease. When you compare the costs of the 19 and younger group with the productivity of older people working longer, it gives a big boost to the gross domestic product (GDP).

U.S. POPULATION
CHANGE BY GENERATION

Age Group	Population in 2020 (millions)	Population in 2050 (millions)	Difference in Population (millions)	Percentage Change
0–39	173.2	182.4	9.2	5.3
40–79	147.8	185	37.2	25.7
80+	12.6	81.7	69.1	548

Where we depart from lower forecasts is not in their assumptions about birth rates or immigration, but rather in the third component of population growth: death rates. Most simply stated, if death rates have been falling *without* the assistance of the genetic discoveries like those described in this book (as well as many others that will occur as others stand on the shoulders of these giants for the next 30 years), imagine the declines in death rates that will occur as the Great Age Reboot sets in.

For example, changing white fat to brown fat holds the promise of making obesity a problem of the past. This would eliminate most deaths associated with obesity-related disease. That alone would make the typical person's Reboot age 20 years younger than their RealAge at age 75 (not to mention what it would do to the one-trillion-dollar-plus diet industry). Unthinkable to eliminate obesity-related diseases? Remember that it was once unthinkable that measles, mumps, chicken pox, and polio would be eliminated. Yet now most people under the age of 40 have no concept of these once common killers.

The prospect of longer life expectancy for children and young adults is invariably greeted as a great social victory (for all but the most devoted Malthusians, who have never been right) as people grasp that younger generations will be productive for many years to come. They will recognize that the opportunity of creating large amounts of productive *human capital* is extremely valuable to society (although some members of this cohort will be social burdens for longer periods). The same is true for older ages as well. Bottom line: A larger workforce that works longer doesn't just benefit working individuals, but also society at large—with a massive boost to the economy. This is true whether they are young or *yold*.

As life expectancy increases, it naturally increases income as more (and more productive) people work and innovate. This in turn raises the wealth of individuals and of society. For starters, improved health (whether achieved by healthier living, medical and pharmaceutical improvements, or targeted genetic and epigenetic engineering) allows each worker more working days, thereby increasing the GDP. For example:

- Just one more working day a year per worker today in the U.S. due to improved health increases the GDP by about $90 billion annually and generates $15 billion in federal tax revenues.

- The present value of this annual savings of one day more per person into perpetuity reveals a societal wealth gain of roughly $3.6 trillion and $610 billion in additional tax revenue. And this is just for an extra day; imagine extra weeks, months, years, and even decades.[4] Moreover, the considerable economic benefits we attribute to each additional year of longevity are conservative, compared with estimates by Andrew Scott, Martin Ellison, and David Sinclair that put that number at $38 trillion per additional year.[5] These dual projections reveal longevity as an advantage for both individuals and society at large.

Such incremental longevity income will pay for many important priorities, including medical services and retirement benefits. In addition, greater health reduces medical outlays, which reduces the cost burden of aging. That is, increased health increases the stock of human capital, which in turn generates enormous income and wealth and reduces health care outlays, not to mention allowing additional quality time with our loved ones. As the number of workers rises so do the income benefits and savings.

| | | | | |

Even as many have chosen lifestyles that promote epigenetic changes that increase chronic disease, the population as a whole has increased longevity by 2.5 years every 10 years since 1880 (see Chapter 1). And data from the Cleveland Clinic indicates that large swaths of working populations can be incentivized to make healthier choices (see page 185). Furthermore, the treatments we've described (and others) are likely to be available to all, so most people will be able to be younger—maybe not as young as if they had made a few healthier choices earlier in life but younger enough to be productive for many years, and to greatly reduce health care costs. If more employers, as well as Medicaid and Medicare programs, adopted such incentive programs, the medical cost savings would be huge.

But the gains made by an extra healthy day each year are small potatoes compared to the gains derived from the collective power of 124 million people now working five to 10 years longer. And by 2050, the number of productive people working longer will be substantially greater than 124 million. Plus, this additional cohort will skew older—an advantage for federal, state, and local government expenses, since those under 21 require schooling and educational outlays while those older than that are more likely to be paying Social Security, Medicare, and state and federal taxes.

People frequently point to the supposed "fiscal burden" of an older population as if it is a reason that people should die when they hit 65. But this is an absurd mindset for many reasons. First, these people have earned the right to some degree of public support in retirement for their many years of financially supporting previous generations. It would be intergenerational theft for these people to lose the benefits they have earned and paid for honestly over their long lives.

In addition, many continue to work well after 65, in which case they are continued "fiscal surpluses." And these fiscal-surplus years will grow dramatically over the next 30 years.

While these rebooted seniors will have more retirement years, they will have earned their keep by having supported previous generations longer.

Another factor is that there are huge "fiscal deficits" associated with youth, and yet no one seriously suggests that this is a reason to eliminate children. Children are financial burdens in their early years (which now often stretch well into their 20s). But people understand that they eventually become productive fiscal contributors. And as the young become a smaller share of the population, the "fiscal burden" of youth will fall as a share of the GDP. How much do children cost? A lot. A recent U.S. Department of Agriculture report estimates costs of $12,000 to $14,000 per child per year for ages one through 17. Add to this about $35,000 a year for each year of university tuition and room and board for those who go on to college. Plus, their insurance, cars, vacations, and electronic devices (not to mention seemingly unending phone, Netflix, and Spotify bills) and various child-focused social programs. All told, it is likely that each child imposes a fiscal deficit of $300,000 to $500,000. As children are less prevalent, the money saved on these costs will be directed elsewhere, including to supporting retirees.

To give you a sense of how this would play out in practice, if each worker 55 and older today were to work just one year longer due to improved health over the next 10 years, it would increase the GDP by $340 billion (about 1.5 percent) annually. That's $340 billion more than anticipated—and that's just for one year. As a result, federal government revenues would rise by $57.8 billion annually, while state and local government revenues would rise by $34 billion each year. The present value of this gain is a $13.6 trillion GDP increase, a federal revenue increase of $2.3 trillion, and state and local government revenue increases of $1.4 trillion.

That is, working just a year longer generates a societal wealth windfall equal to about 65 percent of the current GDP. And it is likely that work lives will be extended five years because of 10- to 20-year extensions in healthy lives. A five-year increase in work life for all workers generates an additional $1.7 trillion (8 percent of GDP) annually. (Remember, by 2050, the number of productive people working longer will be substantially greater than 125 million.) And if in 2050, workers living to age 100-plus decide to work an additional 10 to 20 years (making 75 to 85 the typical retirement age), the additional output and wealth generated is truly mind-boggling! Further, the reduced percentage of the population that needs to be supported until after their education is complete would decline by about 24 percent (from 25 percent under age 19 to 19 percent).

The point to stress is that we believe people will work 15 to 20 more highly productive years as the Great Age Reboot kicks in. These extra years plus reduced youth costs plus a 117.5 million population increase plus massively lower costs associated with chronic diseases and ever increasing productivity over the next 30 years will easily pay for added years.

Of course, society will need to raise the age of qualification for Social Security and Medicare (or their equivalents) accordingly; to fail to do so would be like having benefit eligibility at age 40 today. It will not happen overnight, but it will happen by grandfathering eligibility. Society will adjust. It always has.

After all, society will have plenty of both income and wealth to cover future obligations. The real problem is the sticky political issue that everyone wants someone else to pay. But this is what politics is all about. And as long as there are ample resources, politicians will decide the allocation of these burdens. Examples from the past include changing the retirement age (hardly etched in stone), the tax rate, the phase-out level for FICA taxes, beneficiary policies, indexation of benefits, etc. These areas, not the availability of societal resources, will be the battlegrounds.

Such increases in work life are not flights of fancy. Seventy years ago, people who lacked retirement savings worked well into their 70s if they lived that long. This was in spite of jobs being far more physically demanding. In other words, "retirement" is a recent state. Since 1992, the labor force participation rates of those 65 to 69 have risen steadily from 20.6 percent to 38.3 percent.[6] This is in marked contrast to all younger age categories, which have experienced flat to falling labor force participation rates over this period. Not surprisingly, many surveys show that the main reasons people give for working after age 64 are social connectivity, relationship building and maintaining, and to have additional spending power.[7]

Similarly, the workforce participation rates of those 70 to 74 have risen from 11.1 percent to 24 percent over this period, while those over 75 increased from 4.5 percent to 10.5 percent. These increases are registered across all levels of education but are most pronounced among college graduates. That is to say, society's high earners are the most likely to extend their work lives (and most have now learned how to work from home). They not only produce; they continue to pay into Social Security, private pension plans, and taxes. They will be extending their prime years.

These numbers demonstrate that we can absolutely afford an aging society. In fact, enhanced longevity is *essential for our society*. That's because if longevity increases without better health, it will mean higher costs of medicine and health care as people live longer. And that financial burden can overwhelm a country's ability to handle an aging and unhealthy demographic. It's not just about longevity, but about *healthier* longevity.

As observed earlier in the book, every developed country will be challenged to provide the current standard of living and medical expenses if they do not increase healthy and productive longevity.

In fact, we think the savings for societies engendered by longevity reboots can be much greater than we have stated. Instead of just keeping the percent of GDP spent on medical costs at the level it is now, there are likely to be much more substantial savings. We intentionally underestimated the savings, as we do not know which of the advances will come to fruition—just that one or more will.

Enhanced longevity is essential for civilization. In every society in the past, the greatest association with societal and personal GDP increases is longevity—even much greater than schooling. And if we use these extra resources wisely, we can afford longer and healthier lives. (In fact, if we are going to live 25 or more healthy years, it would make sense that we'd choose to work an extra five to 15 years.)

These numbers also demonstrate that we must embrace a

revitalized lifestyle to live in a society with improved health and growing longevity. Increased longevity is synonymous with increased GDP from increased human capital: the real wealth of the nation. Increased longevity also will go a long way to offset declining birth rates, with aged workers in their prime working years longer, high-earning years generating income which more than offsets the projected lower percentage of the total workforce of lower-income, younger citizens contributing to Social Security and paying taxes.

The Price of Longevity

If real per capita GDP grows by just 1.5 percent a year through 2050 (less than the historic norm), it will generate an additional $36,000 a year in real purchasing power per person by the end of this period: $100,000 versus a total of $64,000 today (1.5 percent greater than inflation compounded annually). That means that on average, every year between now and 2050, per capita real GDP will be notably higher than it is today (as has been the case in the past), representing discretionary real income far above and beyond today's needs.

Believe it or not, the present value of this real income increase is $1.9 million per person. This huge discretionary increase will fund both consumer spending and retirement savings, as well as social support programs, along with Social Security, outlays to support economic dislocation like the CARES and RECOVERY Acts during the coronavirus pandemic, and Medicare.

In addition, as improved health simply delays the cost burden of ill health, it provides more time for real growth to buffer the cost of the final (expensive) years of aging. For example, it is estimated that 8.5 percent of total U.S. medical spending (which amounts to roughly 18 percent of the GDP) is for the final year of life. And 16.7 percent of all health care spending occurs in the final three years of life. This means that $323 billion is currently spent on people in their final year, and $635 billion on those in their final three years. Most of that is for hospital care, with additional amounts for long-term care and other related services.

If improved health delays when these "final" three-year outlays occur by 20 years, money that would otherwise have been spent on sick people can instead be used in more productive and enjoyable ways (there's no decrement in health care costs, just a flattening of the curve—that is, the health care economy stays level or just increases at the rate of growth of the economy rather than increasing at three to four times that rate as it has in the past two decades). If we delay for five years $30 billion of medical spending a year, society receives a present gain of $10 trillion. This is best understood by imagining what their return would be if people took the money they would have spent on medical outlays and invested it in a diverse stock portfolio. If you get five extra years of lower health care costs, that's more money to keep and more that can grow through compounding. Spending less on health for even five extra years allows for exponential growth of the money that is saved. Simply stated, it is better to spend later than today. The point to grasp is that the economic benefit of delaying ill health is huge. Delaying medical costs for the individual means that we not only would have the money we would otherwise have spent but also would have five years of compound earnings on this amount. At a societal level, it is best thought of as having five more years of productive output from those individuals, making seniors not only affordable, but also a huge social asset. In addition, our extended lives will fuel demand for goods and services, driving economic growth. And most important, of course, we will have more time with our loved ones.

In addition, because an estimated 75 to 80 percent of all medical outlays are for lifestyle-related diseases, taking voluntary lifestyle steps to live more healthfully dramatically reduces medical costs.[8] Even if only 40 percent of the population adopts healthier habits, there would be a roughly 25 percent drop in medical outlays, or $950 billion annually in the U.S. This represents a staggering 4.5 percent of GDP saved each year simply through healthier lifestyles! Every year!

Think about what a $1 trillion yearly decline in medical outlays would achieve. Consensus doomsday models show that by 2027, medical costs will rise from $3.7 trillion to about $5.9 trillion yearly of a $30.6 trillion (nominal) GDP. At that time, medical outlays in the U.S. (and we've exported our habits and costs to all other developed countries) are generally projected to grow to 19.4 percent of GDP (these costs may already be there in 2021). This represents a per capita outlay increase from roughly $11,000 in 2019 to $17,000 in 2027. But if just 40 percent of the U.S. population implements self-engineered genetic and epigenetic resets via lifestyle management, it will save about 5 percent of GDP ($1.5 trillion a year) by 2027 (see pages 132–33). Still an increase in the health care economy but one that is about the same as or less than the growth in GDP.

This savings is very possible—remember, our genes haven't changed since 6 to 8 percent of GDP was spent on medical care in the 1970s. But our lifestyle choices have, and that has increased the incidence and presence of chronic disease.

| | | | | |

All of this will make for a truly radical Great Age Reboot—and you are in control of most of the outcome. Moreover, as less money is absorbed by medical costs and more people begin to work longer and healthily, the hand-wringing about shortfalls in private and municipal and state pensions, Medicare, and Social Security (or their equivalents) should disappear.

There is, of course, a cloudier side of increased longevity. While the benefits of wise decisions grow, the costs of unwise decisions also grow. This dichotomy will create greater disparities in health, income, and wealth if we do not address it over time. The longer we live, the more the decisions we have made regarding our work, savings, and health compound the advantages and disadvantages we experience in our later years.

Personal Economics: The Power of Compounding

How will you personally be able to pay for a longer and younger life? It comes down to two concepts: extending your ever rising earning power by being physically capable of working longer and taking advantage of the amazing power of compounding savings. We've already addressed point one, so let's take a closer look at the power of saving and compounding—and why it's the key to making sure you're financially secure for the Great Age Reboot.

If at the age of 25 you start saving 3 percent of your income every year in a diversified portfolio generating a 5 percent annual return, which you will not touch until a timely retirement, predictions and models indicate that you will be financially OK by the time you retire.

With this 5 percent compounded annual investment return, an extra decade of life results in a 1.6-time increase in your wealth; 20 additional years results in a 2.7-time increase. A further 10 years increases your net worth yet again to a 4.3-time multiple.

The magnitudes in wealth differentials are staggering. It means increased life expectancy can lead to increased wealth inequality between those who save and those who don't. Consider this case study, which beautifully illustrates the power of compounding:

Imagine that at age 25 you earn $30,000 (a modest $15 per hour) and save $900 (3 percent of earnings) annually. At an assumed 5 percent rate of return, that initial nest egg of $900 with no additional contributions grows to $27,384 by the time you are 95. If you make it to 115 and leave it untouched, that amount increases to $72,657. This wealth is all derived from just $900 (3 percent of a very modest income) saved early and invested at a conservative rate of return for all of your life.

If you save 3 percent every year on an income that rises by 4 percent annually (1.5 percent real growth plus 2.5 percent inflation), the compounding of your savings means that:

- By age 35, your accumulated wealth is $15,380.
- At age 45, your wealth is $45,648.
- By age 65, your wealth is $215,903, growing to a stunning $1.4 million at age 95.

By age 70, your original investment generates an average of $1.60 for every dollar you save. All of this can be achieved by rather modest savings and investment returns. Of course, saving 6 percent every year is an even better target than 3 percent, particularly if your employer will match your 3 percent. If you save twice as much each year, you will have twice as much as each dollar saved begets—an additional $1.60 in investment return through age 70. Or, to be specific, you'd have $431,806 by age 65 and $2.8 million by age 95. The key is that saving and patient investment are not just for "rich" people if you are able to start early enough.

This illustration underscores the importance of saving early and often (and even finding an employer with a savings-match program). It may sound basic, but saving is like healthy eating and exercise: You can't start too soon, and when in doubt, do more of it. Also, keep in mind that you don't need to be an investment genius. Just invest in a mutual fund or index fund of broadly diversified stocks and bonds. Be consistent and patient, ideally through automatic deductions each pay period, and never be a panic seller or momentum buyer who tries to beat the market. And if your employer offers to match your contribution, definitely save more.

Investing your savings with patience and pragmatism is like managing stress and choosing a healthy diet. By the same token, not saving or making panicked investment decisions is as deadly to your long-term financial health as obesity or smoking is to your physical health. Just as you do not need to be an Olympic marathoner, you do not need a brilliant hedge fund manager to be realistically financially prepared for your longer, younger life. An important policy question to consider is whether the U.S. can foster wiser investment strategies by introducing mandatory savings plans similar to those in Singapore, Australia, and Holland. These forced-savings programs are attractive because the failure of individuals to save throughout their lives imposes a burden on the rest of society. A forced-savings program decreases wealth and income inequalities among the retired and reduces the incentive for people to spend everything they have and take a free ride on savers. In fact, the savings program sketched out above serves as a broad outline for a mandatory savings program to better prepare people for retirement. While each forced-savings program is unique, in essence they require that 3 to 15 percent of every dollar earned goes into a tax-deferred retirement account managed by investment professionals subject to regulatory oversight and reporting. The savings built up over a working lifetime become available at a governmentally established retirement age. These programs ensure that if you have saved money early and often, your retirement will be much easier to enjoy.

The Inheritance Boom

Over the next 30 years, there will be a great inheritance wave that will provide younger generations with unprecedented resources with which to support both themselves and the older generations. It is estimated that over this period, those dying will transfer $25 trillion to $40 trillion (net of estate taxes) to their heirs.[9] This amounts to these aged citizens retrospectively paying for their social costs while aging, and a whole lot more. We bet that this number further grows but will be delayed in transfer as boomers stay younger and healthier than currently expected. As a point of reference, total outstanding net federal debt was about $16 trillion BC-19 (Before COVID-19) and is now about $24 trillion, meaning that legacy inheritances still more than cover the nation's entire outstanding federal debt.

| CHAPTER 10 |

NEW HEIGHTS FOR HEALTH

Build a better body and brain to experience the effects of a Great Age Reboot

I t's one thing to think about how all of these medical advances could work. It's another when you start thinking about how they actually do work in practice. How will they affect your body? How will they affect your body parts? What can go better and what can go wrong?

In this chapter, we'll take a part-by-part look at your body and what the Great Age Reboot may mean for you as you prepare some of the specific systems in your body for rebooting.

Your Brain

All of the organs of the human body must function well in order for you to live a healthy and full life. But the brain—as the computer of your entire body—is the most essential.

Most of the advances in the area of memory loss and brain-related illnesses relate to diagnosis—that is, knowing you're at risk of memory problems up to 10 years before you even see symptoms. In our experience, memory loss is the most feared condition associated with aging. Many people say they can cope with other "hard" diseases, like heart disease and joint deterioration. But it scares the pudding out of them to consider what it might be like to not remember what was said a second ago—or worse, the faces of their loved ones. This is why many say they don't want to live to 100-plus.

But the quest to preserve your brain is not just about avoiding something that's scary. It's also about preserving and extending youth, and youthful curiosity, learning, playfulness, and relationship building.

Weighing just three pounds, the brain holds some 100 billion neurons—the brain cells that populate your life with memories, feelings, decisions, and thoughts (of which you have some 20,000 a day). Can you wrap your head around the number 100 billion—let alone 100 billion of anything fitting into the size of a medium melon? (For perspective, 100 billion pennies stacked atop one another would stretch to the height of three and a half Mount Everests!)

Ironically, modern medicine still doesn't know that much about the brain, although it is the originator of every advancement known to humanity.

While science has made astronomical advances in understanding neurological function and disease, the brain remains mysterious when it comes to issues of aging and preservation. And that's not even bringing in the concept of artificial intelligence. Will our brains become better because AI can take care of some tasks, allowing our brains to concentrate on others? Or will our brains decrease in power as we rely on other systems to do the work for us? Will new advances allow us to have more power, more creativity, more intellect? Right now, it's hard to say (especially since most research today focuses on stopping age-related decline of brain function).

A quick primer about brain function: Just as your home receives electricity from a main source via power lines, your brain cells receive messages that are transmitted from one neuron to another. When the weather is good, the messages come through loud and clear, and you have no disruption of power. But what happens when storms occur?

In the brain, a storm comes in the form of gunk, or plaque, that builds up to interfere with the connection of cells. That plaque comes from brain waste (yes, all organs have waste). Some of it is called tau protein; some is called beta-amyloid, or sometimes limbic-predominant age-related TDP-43.[1] Essentially, this cell waste attracts inflammation; the buildup disrupts the brain's connections by gobbling them up and reducing their size, as a storm tangles tree branches and makes power lines ineffective.

That becomes a double whammy to our brain: We build up the plaques that cause problems through unhealthy choices, and we're not able to clear them out. Instead, they get gobbled up due to inflammation—which leads to dementia.

The good news: We have mechanisms to help. In the body, the lymphatic system, which you are likely familiar with, clears waste and toxins out through the lungs and other waste-disposal organs (which we're certain you're quite familiar with). In the brain, there's a similar system called the glia-lymphatic system (really glymphatic but let's use glia-lymphatic as we think it describes the system better).[2] But often we don't have optimal ability to clear waste from that area. Not surprisingly, this circumstance is largely related to the food we eat, how much exercise we get, and other lifestyle choices we make, especially regarding sleep.

As you sleep and do not take in water, you become very slightly dehydrated and your brain shrinks a little. Your brain cells shrink more as you sleep longer, making the spaces between your brain cells (your glia-lymphatic pathways) a little bigger, which is key for getting rid of your brain poop. That means the sixth and seventh hours of sleep are key to getting rid of waste and decreasing inflammation that would otherwise destroy brain connections and functioning—including the ability to make new memories.[3]

Unfortunately, nothing—so far—has been proved to reverse Alzheimer's and most related cognitive-dysfunction diseases, despite the fact that there have been more than 140 trials in the last 15 years.

Researchers have been looking at a variety of mechanisms to help slow, stop, reverse, and prevent the damage that happens with memory disorders, and we don't expect this quest to stop. It remains one of the major frontiers in medicine. For example, consider these advances and trials that are already under way:

- Drugs are in the works to help target specific actions happening in the brain. For example, some are aimed at clearing the brain of plaques, while others are intended to prevent the plaques from building up in the first place. Some of the drugs are designed to work in conjunction with the immune system to assist in the process that recognizes and removes toxic substances.

- Some researchers are studying ways to replace damaged neurons, which occur with Parkinson's disease. That's a difficult process; researchers are looking at using collagen—the structural protein in such places as your skin—to help support transplanted neurons.[4]

- The AMBAR study showed in humans that a plasma exchange could help slow cognitive decline (by 50 percent) and maybe even reverse some of the deficits in early dementia.[5] That is a wow-wow-wow if it is repeated, as the plasma exchange process is FDA approved already for other diseases. This is really the first process demonstrated to reverse or slow such decline so substantially that is FDA approved and validated in randomized controlled studies. The process would require an early diagnosis of dementia, however, to be able to be widely employed.

- And many advances are being made in the area of early diagnosis of dementia, as researchers are looking for markers to determine risk long before symptoms show.[6] The hope is that early detection (before neuron destruction) can help slow the progression of the disease through other interventions; you may be able to stop the disease much more readily if treatment begins early. That is, researchers are working on blood tests that could help identify dementia before symptoms show, maybe even five to seven years beforehand.[7] This would make for a more cost-effective way to identify dementia (compared to expensive ways like scans of the brain or spinal taps). Most important, it would give people a chance to slow the progress or even stop the disease through lifestyle interventions. Others are looking at subtle tests of cognitive function for early diagnosis. One Cleveland Clinic start-up company has found a method that predicts cognitive decline 20 years before it becomes clinically evident.

But even as these issues are being explored, we're still far away from a systematic stoppage, much less a reversal and elimination of Alzheimer's and related diseases. Therefore, it's vital for you to use that great gift of free will to help prevent them. The choices detailed on these pages will allow you to implement lifestyle choices that improve your odds of slowing or preventing the onset of brain dysfunction.

Your Immune System

When it comes to your health and longevity, there's a good chance that your immune system is at the top of your mind. And it certainly is at the forefront of discussion when we think about one of the world's most powerful enemies of longevity: cancer, as related in Chapter 6. And this, in many ways, is paramount to our individual and collective futures: getting our defense systems to work better, longer, and stronger.

You know all about defense systems. They're all around us. We have passcodes on our phones and computers. We have locks on our doors. We have guard dogs, safety deposit boxes, alarm systems, remote watching and door monitoring systems, and PINs.

Defense is a priority in today's society. And it's not just because there are evil people out there who would be more than happy to find a one-click-away scheme to siphon thousands from your bank account, or make you pay a ransom to get access to it. It's also because, simply, we want to be able to enjoy for now and the future what is most valuable to us—whether it's our family, our money, our property, or our email accounts.

The most fortified defense mechanism in your body—your immune system—is a highly organized and mobile unit.

We see this defense system in action all the time. It's what rushes in when you scrape yourself. It's what makes you cough and sneeze and torpedo phlegm when you catch a nasty bug. It's what makes your ankle swell when you twist it. Ultimately, it's what heals you.

Yet when we talk about vibrant longevity, it's not just about how your body handles the usual cold or a bum joint. It's much more about how your immune system handles the major threats that can—if not defeated—literally kill you.

This is most obviously on display with deadly diseases.

As we discussed in Chapter 6, scientists are working around the clock to figure out how to eradicate the complex and ever changing disease variations of cancer.

Your body's defense system has many levels of protections and biological roles. And sadly, there are thugs in this world that want to invade and destroy your cells (or better yet, live in them and wreak havoc as they multiply—i.e., SARS-CoV-2, the virus that causes the disease known as COVID-19.)

Your defenses want to ID these punks, fight them if necessary, and banish them from your body to restore order in your biological society.

Why your immune system slowly declines after age 50 remains unclear; maybe it gets less aggressive as we age so as not to attack our own mutated tissues and cause an auto-immune disease. Later in life, the immune system may make mistakes and, as all your cells change due to errors acquired during life, is more prone to attacking its own cells.[8]

The elderly tend to get fewer colds than kids, even though they have a weakened immune system. This happens because our systems develop defenses against antigens; we acquire antibodies to the germs we've defeated in the past (stored in plasma cells in your bone marrow, as mentioned earlier in Chapter 6), and destroy those antigens and viruses before they can multiply and cause that illness.

Some of the ways that the immune system ages:

- *Organs shrink.* The thymus begins to shrink when we are young adults. By middle age, it's only about 15 percent of its maximum size. Adding growth hormone (recombinant) may revive your thymus and decrease immune system aging. But that solution is complex because recombinant growth hormone has other effects than just decreasing thymic aging.[9]

- *Efficiency diminishes.* Although the number of T cells doesn't decrease with aging, T-cell efficiency does decrease. This causes parts of the immune system to weaken.

- *Fighters lose power.* Macrophages, the white blood cells that ingest antigens, don't work as quickly when you age. This slowdown may be one reason that cancer is more common among older people.

- *Defenses weaken.* A decrease in white blood B cells that are able to respond to a new antigen means that the body is less able to remember and defend itself. These changes may partly explain why pneumonia and most forms of infection are more common among older people and cause death more often—and why vaccines are less effective in older people.

Your Heart and Arterial System

Heart and arterial aging problems are the cause of 40 percent of deaths now, and much of what we do about extending longevity will continue to revolve around preserving the heart.[10] New developments will center on improving the technology for treatment and diagnostics to detect issues.

We have already experienced incredible advances in treatments for heart problems—and they undoubtedly have extended lives. Before we look too far forward, it's revealing to see what's been done to lay the foundation for future treatments and advances. Before the 1960s, having a heart attack was very common (and fully half of heart attack victims died within hours). So, while a heart attack in the 1960s was frequently a death sentence, much has changed since then.

One example is medication for controlling blood pressure. In the 1950s, co-author Albert's mother was put on a "white rice only" diet to control her high blood pressure. Her BP did in fact improve, but it was a miserable diet.[11] But that was all we had until the late '50s and early '60s, when there were continuing improvements in medicine.

We now know for sure that a diet rich in simple sugars and foods with saturated fats and their accompanying amino acids (it is what accompanies the saturated fats that we now know makes saturated fat consumption so aging) is one of the main causes of aging arteries, and we have low-sugar, plant-based diets with healthy fats to help prevent arterial aging and diets largely without fats to reverse it.[12]

Now we have more than 150 approved medications to treat high blood pressure and aim for readings under 125 systolic and under 85 diastolic.[13] While BP medications were first used to keep people who had had heart attacks or strokes from having recurrent ones, they quickly evolved into preventive therapies.

And the news only gets better. Other lifesaving interventions for heart attacks include:

- Defibrillators to shock a heart in a lethal electrical rhythm into one that lets you live.
- Pacemakers to kick-start a malfunctioning electrical system.*
- Diagnostics like EKGs to detect an abnormal heart rhythm and pulse oximeters to detect a lack of blood oxygen before it becomes fatal.
- Surgeries to clear arterial blockages (open bypasses, then angioplasties, then stents).**

---

* This technique and that of defibrillation were discovered by cardiology pioneer Paul Zoll. During World War II, Zoll was assigned to a medical unit in Great Britain. One day, he was helping a colleague sew a hole in a shrapnel victim lying on a rug in a makeshift hospital. When the surgeon asked him to put his finger on the injured person's stilled heart so that the surgeon could close the hole, Zoll shuffled his feet on the rug. The static electricity generated from Zoll's shuffle to the on-the-floor victim jumped from his finger to the heart and restarted its electrical pattern, causing the heart to contract. The Zoll medical corporation was born, and is still a major innovator in pacemaker and defibrillator development. (Zoll was one of Dr. Mike's attending physicians in 1971, and shared the story.)

** In 1960 the Vineburg procedure—opening the chest and placing an artery

- Medication. Today, we have medications that allow for greater blood flow and decreased inflammation.
- Valve repair (discussed on page 118).

Just because the inspiring medical advances of today are capable of repairing various ailments does not mean that's all we need to do.

Ultimately, your heart's main job is to deliver nutrient-rich blood through the body, as well as to remove waste. When working well, your heart "pumps." Blood gets shuttled throughout your body via the cardiovascular system of blood vessels. In its prime, this system is a well-functioning machine, ensuring a smooth flow of blood through the heart and vessels, making deliveries to all of your organs.

But that delivery system doesn't always run smoothly. Sometimes, there are obstructions, roadblocks, and detours that cause the system to work less efficiently—or not at all. These come in the form of blood sugar and oxidized LDL cholesterol, apolipoprotein B, as well as the increased blood pressure, plaque, and inflammation that's associated with them. When these enemies become too overwhelming, your body's GAME OVER sign turns on.

When blood flow is slow or obstructed, oxygen can't get

---

into the sac surrounding the heart—was found useless by a randomized trial that showed sawing open the breastbone was as effective as the Vineburg was at relieving heart pain. That led to radiologist Mason Sones inventing coronary arteriography at the Cleveland Clinic to define the anatomy of the arteries that supply blood to the heart (we're told he did the first angiogram while smoking a cigarette).[14] That then led to the development of coronary bypass surgery. And then to the development of a balloon on the end of a catheter to dilate the area of narrowing in coronary arteries; and now to wire mesh to stent arteries that have been dilated open.

to your vital organs as effectively (or at all). Over time, if the obstruction is large enough, the cutoff of blood flow can cause heart attacks, strokes, and other vascular issues. And without proper flow, the damage to organs and systems can ultimately lead to organ dysfunction or failure. That includes your heart; if blood doesn't feed the heart for even a few minutes, the cells of the muscle that tries to work all the time become damaged and soon die.

This is why it's so important to get to a hospital fast in the case of a heart attack. The procedures in use today open up the blood vessels to save marginal cells and to allow the signals from dying cells to call forth stem cells and growth factors that will become and develop heart cells over the next six weeks.[15] These new cells grow into functioning heart muscle cells and increase contractile power and squeeze more blood out of the left ventricle. The ejection fraction—the fraction of blood in the left ventricle that is ejected—increases from about 15 to 25 percent on day one after a heart attack to 55 to 65 percent six weeks later. And you feel energetic again. But if the stem cells do not make it to the injury in time or are not nourished by the right form and amount of stimuli and growth factors (from exosomes of some stem cells or maybe dying cells), then new heart cells are not formed and the heart muscle cannot eject as much blood. You form a fibrous scab where the muscle cells should be contracting. Or if the heart cells cannot relax as well as they should (that's when your muscles use energy, in relaxing to allow for a more vigorous contraction), then you develop what is called diastolic dysfunction and eventually heart failure. You can't fill the heart with enough blood to eject enough to supply the rest of the body.[16]

Repairing hearts is the promise of stem cell and growth factor (exosome) treatment as described in Chapter 3—to cut out the scars and replace them with new muscle cells that contract in unison with the existing heart muscle cells so your heart muscle can eject blood to the rest of the body with a normal (55 percent or greater) ejection fraction. And while treatments with these therapies have been the promise since 2000 or so, we are just now beginning to see the rigorous trials needed to make sure that if such treatment works it is available widely by 2030 or so. That means doing what you can for yourself now is essential so you can make it to the time when your heart will be able to benefit from these new longevity disruptors.

Your Joints, Muscles, and Bones

When it comes to our physical infrastructure, we *do* have replacement parts. We can replace hips and knees, for example. We can repair torn soft tissues, like ligaments and tendons, and if you count the latest advancements in prosthetics, we can even swap bones for high-tech limbs.

These are some of the best medical advances made to date, normalizing the lives of people who have worn-out parts or are experiencing chronic pain. But some swaps—including those involving your spine, as well as the muscles and nerves intertwined with it— will take a long time to come to fruition.

No doubt, most of us take movement for granted. You want to reach for the almond butter on the top shelf, and your brain just tells your body to do it. You need to go to the bathroom, and you just get up and go. You encounter a zombie in a back alley at midnight, and your muscles start moving to get you the heck out of there.

And while much of what we do in terms of movement is done without much thought (our bodies follow what our brains want us to do), there's a lot that's going on behind the scenes to get your body to do what you want it to do.

For example, you have more than 650 muscles in your body, all of which give you the strength to do the world's work. Muscles are also the centerpiece of one of our more significant health challenges: back pain. Responsible for about 33 million doctor visits in the United States every year, and an estimated 150 to 240 million lost days of work, back pain often stems from problems with musculature and the prescription typically includes self-management (the position you sleep in, the food you eat, stretching and strengthening) rather than an invasive medical treatment.

Which underscores our main point: We do not yet have superb replacement spines, disks, and surrounding muscles—but you can prepare for them, and they are coming. One of the reasons the spine is so complex is because it contains the intersection of the spinal cord and spinal nerves; the spine and the brain are the most complicated parts to replace or reboot because of this intersection. The data on senolytics as presented in Chapter 4 indicates that help for the large causes of back pain may be on the way.

Your bones act as the levers in your body. As living organs, they actually remodel themselves. Bones aren't a solid structure, but more of a matrix, like the Eiffel Tower (which was in fact modeled after bones because they are so strong). Problems occur when the holes in that matrix become too big and the bones get brittle: That's osteoporosis.

Your bones normally resorb (get thinner) and produce

aggregation (build bone thickness) every day. In the past, drug therapy has allowed us to decrease resorption of bone, or increase production of bone. But until fairly recently, every one of these drugs that thicken bone also increased resorption, so they were fighting against themselves. Today, in a brilliant discovery using the genetics of a rare family in Africa that had strong bones, scientists at Amgen isolated and cloned a protein from those family members to make a dual-action drug that both decreases resorption and increases aggregation (romosozumab).[17] This is yet another example of new genetic science combined with the brilliant molecular biology of Big Pharma that will let you live longer younger.

The connection points between bones, your joints, come in a variety of shapes and sizes. Your hip joint, for example, is a ball and socket, different from your knee joint, which works more like a hinge. Why? Because they're constructed differently, depending on what kind of job they have to do. Your hips don't have a lot of flexibility because they're needed for stability to move you through life. Your shoulders, however, tend to have more range of motion and flexibility—meaning your arms can move in a number of different directions.

The biggest challenge with joints is the deterioration that happens to the soft tissues—like cartilage—found within them; this condition is called osteoarthritis. When that happens, you can experience bone-on-bone rubbing, which can produce pain that is all-caps excruciating. You can slow the deterioration with movement that generates lubrication, by decreasing inflammation by managing stress actively, and by choosing foods that love your joints such as omega-3 (algal and fish oils) and omega-9 fatty acids (extra virgin olive oil) and avoiding the food felons we mentioned in Chapter 7. Happily, there have been many medical advances in this area, especially with hip and knee replacements. Same goes for ligament repair: Torn ACLs and Achilles tendons can now be surgically fixed (though the procedures require long recoveries). New developments, like those discussed in Chapter 8, including growth factors and stem cells on a sponge that join the torn ends of the ligament, may radically improve recovery time.[18]

Like cars, our bodies are not made to last forever. Through years of wear and tear, things fray and break down. That's the cost of living. Part of the goal of the Great Age Reboot is to help you slow down (or stop) the inevitable wear-down that comes with aging.

If you can optimize your body now through self-engineering with lifestyle choices, you'll last longer and be prepared to best handle whatever advances become available.

Movement is one of the arenas in which we've seen the most significant advancement. In 1974, for example, there were about 67,000 joint replacements in the United States; in 2019, there were 1.4 million. By 2050, at this current rate, we could see six to seven million a year: an increase of 360 percent (or about 5 percent a year). While not without limitations, joint replacements are an excellent example of how medical advances have massively improved quality of life. Even better and easier for you is the promise soon to come, arresting the aging of joints altogether (see Chapter 4).

Your Senses

When we age, we do take some things for granted. You know,

the everyday functions that are just sort of there in the background, but you don't really pay attention to them—until they go missing. When senses like seeing, hearing, and smelling malfunction, it may not be a life-ender, but it can certainly accelerate cognitive dysfunction and change your life.

What would happen if we could reverse blindness or stop hearing loss by reprogramming cells so that they don't age?

One of our authors, Albert, says that the two greatest health miracles are childbirth and cataract surgery. One brings you into the world; the other lets you see the world clearly once again. Sure, maybe recipients of emergency heart bypass or brain artery stents may suggest that cataract surgery take the number-two spot. But the point is well made: When we think about quality of life, we have to consider the things that make us experience the world around us more effortlessly and richly. And that keep us and our brains stimulated to function well longer. Preserving and restoring eyesight as we get older certainly qualifies. We have seen tremendous progress in the fields of cataract surgery, retinal reattachments, and more.

Now researchers are working on such new advances as epigenetic reprogramming to activate the Yamanaka factors (see page 109) just to the eye and retinal cells, and to specific eye gland cells that decrease the secretion or increase the resorption of fluid. In animal models, this epigenetic reprogramming has reversed the cause of and even state of severe glaucoma.[19] Even more important as we get older is the prevention and reversal of age-related macular degeneration.

THE MOST COMMON PROBLEMS ASSOCIATED WITH EYES AND AGING

Cataract	A cloudy area in the lens that prevents light from passing through to the retina. Large and thick cataracts have to be removed surgically (it's one of the most common surgical procedures in the United States) and replaced with near 20/20 lenses.
Presbyopia	Losing your ability to read the fine print and small type. Welcome to the world of reading glasses.
Glaucoma	A buildup of pressure that can lead to vision loss. It can be treated with everything from medication to surgery, depending on the cause and severity.
Age-Related Macular Degeneration	The macula is the central part of the retina and is made up of nerve cells called cones. Loss of those cells can lead to vision problems.
Dry Eyes	When your tear glands can't produce enough tears, it can lead to itching, burning, and loss of vision.
Retinal Detachment	When the inner and outer layers of the retina separate, it causes vision loss, which can be restored with surgery or laser treatment.

About 30 million injections yearly worldwide just to slow the disease show its prevalence and importance. It is the largest cause of vision loss in the elderly and increases with age from zero percent at age 30 to 10 percent for those over age 80. But researchers may have found a way to keep our retinal cells young and able to see as long as we live. They are inducing autophagy (the cellular self-repair process to get rid of old cells and replace them with younger ones) to stop loss of eyesight in early wet age-related macular degeneration.[20] As mentioned in Chapter 4, a senolytic combo has been found to restore sight in animals with induced wet macular degeneration.[21] Senolytics may also be the go-to breakthrough for reversing blindness from the severe form of macular degeneration.

Imagine stopping sight loss with a senolytic when you are 85, and then reprogramming your eyes and eye muscles so your eyesight is once again as good as it was when you were 20. Mice the equivalent of 100 human years old have regained their 20-year-old sight (in human terms). These therapies were either in late-stage animal testing or early-stage human testing as of late 2020.

Hearing loss is also one of the most common conditions for older adults. As hair cells in the ear decrease with age, so does the ability to hear (this is called presbycusis and can also be the result of exposure to loud noises).

Here's how hearing works: Sound waves hit the skin-like eardrum, which, like any kind of drum, vibrates when hit. That oscillation vibrates the smallest bones in your body, which abut the eardrum, and causes the snail-shaped cochlea (the cavity in the inner ear) next to them to quiver as well.

These vibrations, traveling through fluid in the tubes of the cochlea, stimulate hair cells growing on the insides of these cisterns. Since the hairs are attached to nerves, when they move, the auditory nerves become excited and fire away messages to the brain that allow it to hear the sounds and know what you're listening to. Loud noises—both sudden and cumulative over a period of exposure—cause the fluid to push through the cochlea too aggressively, thus shearing off the hairs. The high-frequency hairs are more vulnerable, making the lost ability to hear higher pitches, including many female voices, one of the sure signs of age-related hearing loss.

Hearing aids and cochlear implants are two foundational technologies that have been able to significantly preserve hearing. And new developments in hearing aids—today, they are more directional, can be controlled by cell phones, and have been radically reduced in price, thanks to Walmart and others—have made them even more effective. And believe it or not, regrowth of hair cells within the ear is in late-stage animal testing (as it happens, the serums that work to restore eyelashes might also work on those hairs in the ear).

The key takeaway for you to keep your sense of hearing young: Hearing loss isn't just about missing out on the sweet sound of waves crashing or choirs singing. There are significant long-term health implications as well. New research shows that decreased hearing is associated with earlier death and more rapid development of dementia.[22]

In a study of 16,000 people, scientists found that a diagnosis of hearing loss between ages of 45 and 65 doubled the chances of a diagnosis of dementia over the next decade or so. And a study from Johns Hopkins University found that older people with hearing loss experienced a cognitive decline up to 40 percent faster than those people who did not.[23]

What's the connection? It's too early to tell if it's biological, but the leading thought is that hearing loss leads to social isolation, which has been shown to be a contributing factor in the development of dementia and aging. But you can reverse this scenario with hearing aids. This opportunity epitomizes the new reality: that you can make healthy lifestyle choices, keep much of your body and brain functioning younger longer, and be prepared for the Great Age Reboot—the regeneration to a much younger you.

PART 4

THE SCIENCE OF SELF-ENGINEERING

Steps you should take today to prepare for the changes of tomorrow

While science will show incredible advances when it comes to extending and improving life, the fact is that we can't rely on everyone else to do the work. We will be better prepared to accept and benefit from these advances the stronger and healthier we are. This is what self-engineering is all about—reprogramming your epigenes to optimize your health and fortify your body.

Over the following decades, you may have dozens of new decisions to make about how to care for your body, but that decision-making should start right now. Begin today to make the lifestyle choices that will best prepare you for the Great Age Reboot. The following chapters will show you how.

CHAPTER 11

DECIDE AND CONQUER

Good decision-making will make or break your reboot

You're no stranger to decisions. Some are habitual (take a shower), and some are easy (yes, you'll take the silo-size black coffee, please), and a few are monumental (move to a new home). But whether the choice is great or small, there's no doubt that your brain spends a fair bit of energy evaluating all kinds of choices.

One of humanity's greatest gifts is free will: the notion that our brains are free to roam and explore, to make what may turn out to be good or poor choices. Free will is what makes us human, and what makes life so damn grand. But that free will is also why heroin or a jelly doughnut may surf their way through your body. So don't let the free will to make one bad decision destroy your ability to make better free-will decisions down the line.

As far as we can tell, the Great Age Reboot is not going to be a one-stop shop. Maybe in 2187, but not in the next 10 or 20 years. Think of a senolytic injection to attack knee arthritis.

Maybe that will help you dance without pain, but this is a one-step-at-a-time process for a while. Maybe you should wait until pain limits your movement more, or maybe the benefit is worth the risk now. We'll take you through the process of understanding the benefits and the risks as they now are known. But the decision is yours. So your decision-making—your free will—will serve as your pilot in achieving a healthier, stronger brain and body, with many excellent years to live in it and the resources to pay for it.

In this chapter, we describe our major principles for making advantageous decisions as they apply to longevity and living a younger, healthier life.

Do-It Decision #1:
Take Control of Your Health and Wealth

We'll tell you a familiar story. Someone you know gets the news of a bad medical diagnosis. There's a tough road ahead, the doctors say. Everyone surrounding that person feels horrible. They huddle around, they try to help, they feel helpless.

But then something happens. The person whose future looked bleak pulls through. While there could be any number of reasons a treatment worked, one of the health professionals will assert that the patient made it because she was in good shape, she was otherwise healthy, and her body and her immune system were strong. And deep down, you know there's truth to it. While a strong body can't weather every medical storm, there's little doubt that a stronger body can surely weather storms better than a weaker one.

That principle is the one that guides us as we think about the Great Age Reboot.

You will be better prepared, more fortified, and have a stronger biological shield if you take control over your health destiny, rather than wait for every fix to come your way. The same holds true for your financial destiny. The stronger you are now, the better prepared you will be for the future.

Why?

There are many unknowns as to our timeline and the availability of these antiaging advances. Will these new advances (brown-fat-from-white-fat transformations, stem-cell regeneration, gene editing, epigenetic reboot, senolytics, autophagy, plaque busting, telomere lengthening, 3D printing, and artificial bolstering of organs and systems) be available and be safe when administered once or many times? How will they get perfected over time? How will your current health status influence your ability to take advantage of these treatments? How will industries change, and what will those changes mean for personal income and retirement? But we know that you can choose to make it much more likely you'll benefit from the changes that do come.

When it comes to your health, your original parts are nature's most masterful design. And if we can keep those parts in their original packaging, there's a good chance that your health outcomes will be even better when you do use rebooting methods.

The reboot shouldn't be about saving your life. It should be about enhancing it.

Your future depends on what you decide now. And those decisions will make you live stronger in both body and pocketbook, and prepared to fully enjoy the Great Age Reboot.

Do-It Decision #2:
Select Your Team

We know life, medicine, and finances can be complicated, nuanced, and trickier than a Vegas magician. You have to be the one to make decisions about what is best for you.

The most important thing you can do is to make sure you build a loving, informed, and loyal team around you. That includes family. That includes friends. And that surely includes a community of trusted experts—everyone from doctors to financial advisers. Why? Because the best decision-making is not just about what you feel in your gut or even read in this book. It's about triangulating several opinions and insights from people who love you—and who may know more than you do.

You may already have a strong team around you. And if so, that's a 10-mile head start. But if you're in the stage where you're still trying to find or develop your own community of advisers, then you need to take some things into consideration, such as:

Trust: This is built over time, for sure. Ultimately—with such decisions about your body and money on the line—you have to know that your team has your best interests in mind.

Knowledge: Does your team know the latest research, understand how to evaluate info, and make smart choices? This isn't always easy to know off the bat, but you'll get a good sense by asking pointed questions.

Honesty: Your team shouldn't simply yes-yes-yes your current view. They should care enough about you to push back, to challenge you, and to say things that you may not want to hear.

You need inquisitive and honest team members who

value information and have your best interests at heart. Your father, mother, siblings, and spouse may love and care about you, but they must also be inquisitive and value information to be helpful with decision-making. And one more thing we believe about your decisions and health: If you are to make a choice that involves doing something for more than three days or has an effect that will last longer than three days, get a second opinion. Remember that at Johns Hopkins University, when biopsy specimens were analyzed by expert academic pathologists, it was determined that cancer was often misdiagnosed.[1] [2] You have to sort your team depending on your decisions, and your team will need to evolve over time as people die or move, as friendships fray, and as new life challenges arise. In the plan in the next chapter, this team will start to curate decisions for you—but you will need an ongoing longevity team to help you decide what and when specific choices are right for you as an individual.

Do-It Decision #3:
Win the Battle Between Brain and Heart

Your body was built to work in harmony. When you eat your salmon (X), it sends out signals to start digestion (Y) and decides how to use those calories for energy (Z). When you see the couch that needs to move across the room (X), your brain tells your muscles to contract (Y), and your legs, core, and shoulders all work to lift that purple-flowered butt warmer (Z).

That's the way it's supposed to work.

Yet every now and then, elements of your body act more like friendly foes—competing *against* each other rather than working *with* each other.

We see that very thing happening when it comes to decision-making. Logic versus love. Need versus want. Reason versus emotion.

There's good reason for this. Evolutionarily, we needed to be able to react with emotion. Controlled by a part of the brain called the amygdala, emotion is very reactive—and because we react quickly to emotion, it allows us to make decisions without even thinking we're making a decision. Makes sense when it comes to survival. (You see something black and slithering in the grass, and you jump out of the way. SNAKE! Better to jump out of the way using our emotion of fear first and later realize that it was a garden hose than to take a few minutes to logically think about it and wind up with a cobra bite on your face.)

Emotional reactions are like that reptilian one: Because they happen quickly, they help us survive.

Of course, we need our brain's help, too; everything can't be decided via a reaction. In our distant past, we needed logic and executive function to figure out how to build shelter and to remember where our camp was after a long day of hunting. That decision-making took longer because processing—which takes place in the frontal lobe of the brain—takes more time neurologically.

Logical reasoning helped us survive.

Fast-forward to our modern era. We still have two forces at work when it comes to making choices: quick, reptilian ones. Longer, executive ones.[3]

Does it make sense sometimes to respect the reptile? Yes, of course. We should let our emotions help direct us. You love what you love because of the way it feels.

But is the emotional, reactive process the best way to make

all decisions? Of course not. And frankly, that's what has gotten us into a whole lot of trouble. We often buy with our eyes, rather than our budget (which is why we have so much debt). We eat with our eyes, rather than following smart dietary guidelines (which is why we have so much fat). And we make decisions that may make us feel better in the short term, but have serious consequences for the long term.

In many ways, it's not our fault. Our bodies are wired to react first; that's why we fall victim to ads from Amazon and goodies from the grocery store, even if we know they're not best for us long-term. In this way, our brain and our heart (really our executive functioning part of the brain and our reptilian brain) do compete when making decisions.

Is there a simple fix for this? Not really, but there is a strategy: indulging in just a little bit of patience. That is, if you can delay your emotional decision—even for just a few minutes in some cases—it will allow you time to let your executive function process the information, weigh the options, and make the very best decision for you.

This comes into play every single day (and at every single meal when it comes to food). It also comes into play when you make spending decisions (what you want right now versus what you can save for the future).

Say you have made a commitment to eating better, maybe losing some weight, and just getting more control over your diet. That's the major, umbrella decision. But tomorrow is book club, and you know what book club means: The wine will be flowing, the fondue will be oozing, and the milk chocolate treats will be within a finger's reach at all times. The emotional reaction: These look good. I like these. Eat these. Yum.

In this case—and in many cases where your health is in play—you just need time to veto your reptilian instincts. It's not always easy; like playing the piano or solving difficult math problems, it takes some practice and some commitment. But it's worth working on—pausing before making a fast decision and really thinking through the benefits and risks.

Do-It Decision #4:
Think It Through

Some people make decisions really quickly (this involves the reptilian brain and is not usually the best way), while others take so long that they become too paralyzed by fear to actually move ahead. Some write down pro-con lists, while others just say what the heck and go for it. But what are the best strategies, according to decision-making experts? These are a few of our favorites.

Ben's pro-con list: Benjamin Franklin had a cool twist on this concept. Instead of just listing pros and cons and seeing which column was longer, he made the lists and assigned some "weight" to each item.[4] He then canceled out items of equal weight—and thus could easily see whether the pros or the cons won out.

Remind yourself of goals: Sometimes, the big picture gets lost when making an in-the-moment decision. When you're making big choices, write down not only the choice, but what your ultimate goal is. See how that goal will be affected by your decision not only now, but also a year into the future. The *Harvard Business Review* also recommends writing down alternatives to your decisions—and what effect those will have on the choice you're making. The *HBR* found that managers who follow a process that includes these steps made faster decisions and saved time doing so.[5]

Clear your mind: Some research shows that it's important to look for the things you missed initially (perhaps because of a subconscious bias toward a certain decision). So when thinking a decision through, try to identify information that you may be missing—the holes in your story. This hearkens back to the point that, in many cases, you need to let your executive function overrule your reptilian response.

Do-It Decision #5:
Customize

What's good for you isn't necessarily good for others—and vice versa. Consider this story: In 1985, a discovery by a major U.S. pharma firm led to a significant success in breast cancer treatment in two animal species. The phase I human trials showed no major safety concerns, but the study failed in phase II. The problem was with the cohort that was used. Half the patients had a gene that failed to metabolize the drug and they developed toxicity; the other half had a gene that metabolized the drug so quickly that it had no effect. When this problem was finally discovered in 2010 after gene sequencing of humans and of their tumors became more common, researchers realized that this beneficial drug had not helped the hundreds of thousands it could have since 1985. The point: The Human Genome Project has led to a better understanding of why something can be bad for some but good for others. That has led to scientific progress that is letting us live younger for longer.

In medicine, customization may turn out to be the prevailing theme when it comes to diagnosis and treatment.[6] But it's also worth applying the same theory to you and your self-care.

In your quest to live healthfully and to save money for the extra years, there are recommended practices. But you also have to be aware that your body, your environments, and your circumstances may be different. And it's OK to tweak, to adjust, to customize decisions to fit *you*. One of the decision processes is to know what your risks and benefits are—and to consider that risk-to-benefit ratio before you make your decision. For example, you should talk through decisions about new technology with your doctor—because the benefits of some may cause other risks depending on how your body works.

CHAPTER 12

SELF-ENGINEERING YOUR FUTURE

The best way to prepare for a healthier future is being healthier now

Take a moment to visualize your favorite place in the world that requires you to walk up an incline. Maybe it's the Spanish Steps in Rome or the Potala Palace in Tibet. Or maybe it's a serene hill in your local park. Or the top row of your favorite team's stadium.

Now, imagine that you've reached the summit. Take a look down at the other folks trekking toward you. You will see two kinds of people.

First, there's the spry set. These are the bouncy beings that kangaroo from the bottom to the top. They're smiling, laughing, barely breaking a sweat, and fully enjoying the journey. They're excited about reaching the destination, and—despite the fact that it took some effort—can't wait to experience what awaits when they arrive. *Lickety split, that was fun.*

Second, there's the group that's struggling. Who have to stop and catch their breath 10 times on the way up.

Every. Step. Takes. So. Much. Out. Of. Them. Huff. Puff. Are. We. There. Yet?

And many refuse to even try.

You're probably more like one of these groups than the other. What's the difference between them, besides the speed and ease at which they travel? It might be their size or age, yes. It's most certainly their overall health. But you know what it's less likely to be? Their genes endowed at birth.

Instead, it's their lifestyle choices. In order to prepare for the Great Age Reboot, you have to be willing to change—not only to get and stay healthy, but to have enough health to repair yourself when repairs are needed. There is certainly a fantastic future ahead. But to enjoy it and relish your longevity, you will need to be a genetic engineer now. The upside? You will literally get to change your family medical destiny—if you want to. This is important, since about 40 percent of premature deaths in the U.S. today are related to lifestyle choices. Lifestyle and genetics are intertwined in that your lifestyle choices influence how those genes function—and thus, how your body functions. That is, your choices determine about 1,200 of the 1,500 genes that are "on" and how your body chooses the other 21,000 that are "off."

Whether you're the one who zips up the incline or struggles to the top, you have self-engineered your body to end up in that place. You influence how your body functions—through the effect your actions have on organs, tissues, fluids, systems, processes, and *everything* that your body does.

Studies of gene expression show that you can turn genes on or off with lifestyle changes. After implementing lifestyle interventions of diet, stress management, and physical activity, men were able to turn off the genes that fostered prostate cancer growth and turn on a gene that produced a protein that causes cancer cells to self-destruct. The same process applies for colon and breast cancer. Lifestyle changes switched on genes that fought cancer—and turned off genes that promoted cancers.[1]

You have the ability to change how your body works and reacts—and ultimately how healthy you are and how long you may live.

That is genetic self-engineering.

You may never have taken a chemistry, biology, physics, or engineering class. And you may have only a vague concept of DNA and cells. Yet you are a supreme genetic engineer who has the power to help determine, on a daily basis, which of thousands of your genes are turned off or on. Each healthy act switches on youth-promoting genes and switches off genes that cause you to age. This process is the result of millions of years of evolution. Good choices (and the proteins that are developed because of them) beget more good proteins, and the activation of bad genes begets more bad and destructive genes being turned on.

This genetic engineering occurs through a lifetime of daily decisions that you make. It occurs because of what you eat today—and what you ate the thousands of days before that. Those choices can make you healthy, which in itself will allow you to repair yourself when the time comes. Therefore, a lifetime of decisions—getting regular exercise or not, smoking or not, handling stress or not—can make the difference between whether you rocket up the incline, slug through it, or completely avoid it.

The top-of-the-steps metaphor is just one way to compare people who fall on the healthy end of the spectrum with those who fall on the other end. But the larger point—whether you're comparing ability to walk up steps, clothes sizes, vim and vigor, or trips to the doctor's office—is that this whole fight for longevity and "youthfulness" is far less about a predetermined genetic destiny than you think. In fact, science tells us that when you are under the age of six, your genes determine what happens, but by the time you are 55, 80 percent of your health outcomes are determined by your choices, which dictate which of your genes are on and which are off.[2] So while your genetic component at birth certainly has some influence on your ultimate health and longevity, life outcomes are much more about engineering via your behaviors, choices, and decisions than they are about genes.

Ultimately, we believe that there are three main reasons your pursuit of optimum health and youth through lifestyle choices is an imperative.

You Should Build a Strong Foundation Now

You probably know someone who has survived a horrific disease, accident, or surgery. One of the main themes that often emerges from these stories is that the person's preexisting physical and mental strength fortified their body for battle and made them better equipped to handle the stresses that they endured.[*] That

---

* That's how RealAge started.[3] For every 10 years younger you are, you decrease your complication rates and risk of death and disability after surgery threefold. So Dr. Mike developed RealAge—the actual age of your body based on the net present value of your health and lifestyle choices and your genetics—to motivate presurgical patients to make choices that made them the equivalent of 10 or more years younger in the two weeks surrounding their major surgery. Surgical out-

is true with the recent pandemic—over 85 percent of the people who required ICU care and an even higher percentage of those who died had one or more of six preexisting conditions (obesity, hypertension, type 2 diabetes, heart disease, chronic lung disease, or immune dysfunction) or was over age 70.[4] That same line of thinking, we postulate, will come into play when we're talking about longevity—that is, a little self-genetic-engineering via healthy choices will help you prevent chronic disease and set you up for longevity. The better your physical shape, the higher the chances that new antiaging procedures will "take" at a high level, with fewer complications. Stronger at the start means you'll be stronger through the entire race and all the way to the finish.

It Is Unclear How Many Reboots You'll Get

Perhaps in a 25th-century world, there will exist some dressing-room-like catacomb that allows you to walk into a booth and erase every cigarette you've smoked, every couch you've potatoed, every potato you've ever fried. But for the foreseeable future, it's more likely that your ability to maximize your reboot chances will depend on your commitment to improving your biology through proven means: nutrition, physical activity, sleep, not smoking, and stress management. These methods provide natural ways of engineering your DNA switches—perhaps not with laser-like precision, but to great effect nonetheless.

---

comes at institutions that employed that strategy, like the University of California at San Francisco, the University of Chicago, and the Cleveland Clinic, became dramatically better than at peer institutions in that period. Some of those outcome improvements may have been due to this preoperative optimization.

No Matter What Happens, Your Brain Needs You

As we've discussed, your brain remains the final biological frontier. So even if science ultimately allows us to correct our cells, genes, and other mechanisms that make our body work, when your brain goes, you will, too. To maximize the promise of a longer-lasting youth, it's imperative that you self-engineer your DNA switches to protect your brain.

The best news is that the steps you can take to do so are the same as those you can take to protect the rest of your body. So when you become committed to making your noggin as good as new, you'll be doing your own DNA reboot. And you can do that every day.

Changes That Work

Let's go back to the car metaphor. Even if you know nothing about engines or spark plugs or transmissions, you know this: Your car is a complex machine with a lot of moving parts. And it is capable of getting you from here to there.

But that car can be the best in class—beautiful, cutting edge, and slick—and it won't mean squat if the driver is reckless. The best-engineered car in the world (your initial genetic setting endowed at birth) will crash if the driver is intoxicated or driving with a blindfold, while a run-of-the-mill car in the hands of a highly skilled driver will make the trip effortlessly.

The five main actions outlined below have been proved to have the most influence over your biological function, and are discussed more thoroughly in the plan in Chapter 13.

Science is about to offer us the Garden of Eden—a chance not just at prolonged life, but at prolonged *youth* or rather (and

HOW YOU CHILL, HOW YOU FRIEND & YOUR PURPOSE IN LIFE	WHAT & WHEN YOU EAT
When stress is high, it triggers a cascade of hormonal effects that make it the number-one ager. It's impossible to eliminate stress, but how you respond to it will dictate the effect it has on your health. Friends and purpose are key to managing stress.[5][6] And it is possible to slap the snot out of stress and win the hormonal battle.	Your fuel triggers biological processes that influence fat storage, insulin production, arterial health, genes that harvest old cells and genes that promote new cell formation, growth hormones (including specific growth hormones for your brain and spinal cord), stem cells, and more. Day in and day out, it's the no. 2 influence[7] on your health (stress is no. 1), as it's the consistent fuel for your cells and systems.
HOW YOU SLEEP	**HOW YOU MOVE**
Sleep is your body's own reset button, as quality and quantity of sleep are crucial to optimum brain health, not to mention optimum energy and minimum fatigue (which is tied to obesity and other health problems).	With major influence over metabolism, bone health, cardiovascular strength, joint health, even brain and other growth and repair factors, and more, being active is a major predictor of longevity (and, on the flip side, inactivity facilitates death and disability).
NOT SMOKING	
Eliminating toxins like cigarette smoke and reducing exposure to other environmental toxins will drastically reduce direct health risks (like dementia, cancer, and heart disease). It will also go a long way in reducing inflammation—a process that ages the body and brain profoundly and relentlessly—as will avoiding other unforced errors (like not washing your hands before eating and texting while driving/walking, which are among those actions that shorten life spans).	

even better) *prolonged youthful years*. But it will be up to you to take advantage of it.

When it comes to self-engineering, you're not going to be—nor does your body expect you to be—perfect all the time. Your longevity depends more on the aggregate of what you do most of the time. You can think about it like any other skill you develop over a lifetime, whether it's shooting free throws, playing piano, or learning a new language. You will miss shots, hit the wrong key, and use the wrong words. But when you practice—and perform the skill consistently—you will be accurate more often than not.

Our goal here is not to tell you to "do this" or "do that"; it's to convince you that you control far more than you think. How can we inspire change? How can we make change? How can we collectively get to better decisions?

We are in a peak period for access to information and have the most medically advanced health industry of all time. And yet two-thirds of Americans are overweight or obese, and millions will die or become ill from choice-related health problems including heart disease, lung cancer, strokes, diabetes, and dementia (yes, the data shows it's possible to reduce more than 60 percent—even 80 percent—of that risk).[8]

Finding the right way to motivate ourselves to make better lifestyle choices is not easy (and we have very effectively exported our bad habits to almost every other developed country). If it were easy, the weight-loss industry wouldn't generate billions of dollars annually, and no one would smoke or vape.

However, we do have some clues about what may work—and what *has* worked.

The questions: Do you want to try—and can you make it work for you?

The Proven Way to Successfully—and Consistently—Make Smart Health Choices

Here's a scenario that plays out over and over: Pat is in good health. Life gets in the way. Pat gains weight. And then a little more. Needs new clothes. Doctors say blood pressure is high. Or LDL cholesterol. Holy crap—Pat needs to do something ASAP or Pat's going to die. Pat starts learning how to cook kale so it tastes great, and loves eating kale. And salmon. And beans. Pat loses weight and feels good. Then life gets in the way again, and damn if Pat feels entitled to a backpack's worth of nachos because of all of the stress. Pat is derailed. Again. Then inspired. Again. Then derailed. Again. Pat is a poor genetic engineer.

And all the while, Pat—and the millions of Americans who yo-yo and struggle and try and cry—is stuck. That's because even if we don't know every nuance about nutrition and exercise, we understand what we need to do. But change is hard. And change hurts. And change isn't always comfortable. So we put our blinders on—we don't see you, CHANGE!—and carry on the best we can.

But if the choices you're making are hurting more than helping, change—and subsequent habits that are the derivation of change—is imperative. There are several factors that are common among people who successfully make positive lifestyle changes:*

---

* In 2008, the Cleveland Clinic, which self-insures its 101,000 employees and their dependents, embarked on a journey to help them get healthier and reduce their and its medical costs. (Dr. Mike served as founding chief wellness officer for the Cleveland Clinic for 12 years and is now emeritus CWO.)

Employees and their adult dependents were given progressively larger financial incentives to reach "6 Normals" and complete two other requirements (see a primary care physician and update their immunizations)—see page 186. In 2018, the incentive was a $1,440 deduction in medical premiums. If their levels continued to stay normal (as substantiated by their primary care practitioner), they got another reduction in premiums each year. The corporate benefit, of course, was avoiding spending millions in direct illness-care and benefit costs. (In the first 10 years, the clinic did not spend $855 million

They strive for these markers. The healthiest bodies are the ones that show "normal" or healthy levels of six key indicators. Mostly, you want to get to "6 Normals + 2"™, which is a barometer for health markers that indicate health success, using the strategies we outline in this section. They include:

- blood pressure of less than 125 mmHg systolic and less than 85 mmHg diastolic
- BMI (a measurement of height-to-weight ratio) of less than 27 or, better, a waist-to-height ratio of 0.40 to 0.55
- fasting blood sugar (associated with diabetes) of less than 106 mg/dL
- LDL cholesterol (a risk factor for heart disease) of less than 70 mg/dL

---

compared with trend and other similar institutions, and the reduced spending is now at over $180 million a year.) Plus, there was better productivity, fewer absentee days, and workers and their families saved over $250 million in premium costs and had notably improved lives.

An important note here is that while the clinic's population was a large one, composed of janitors, clerks, and administrators, as well as nurses and doctors, etc., and medical costs were equal to the national average, it was a population already seemingly interested in health. This is what we would call a study limitation in scientific circles. But you may be surprised to learn that when we began in 2008 only 6 percent of the individuals had what we called "6 Normals +2"™, but 10 years later, 43.6 percent of participants had them. That's truly a remarkable change in the individuals as well as the system. At the Cleveland Clinic today, the cost of health benefits for every employee has experienced only a modest increase since 2008 and costs have been stable since 2013, while in the United States as a whole the average employer cost per employee went up $7,000 per year from 2008 to 2018. If the clinic's system had been replicable for all U.S. workers and Medicare enrollees, it could have saved the country over $1 trillion annually, depending on the level of participation. This clearly underscores the power of self-engineering your DNA switches until external genetic engineering feats—age reboots, new organs, white-to-brown-fat transitions—become available. And this savings at the clinic was achieved with just 43.6 percent of workers and enrollees meeting their Normals. If all workers in the U.S. achieved their Normals, the country's savings would approach $2 trillion annually.

- no cotinine in urine (an indicator of tobacco use)
- completion of a stress management program

Hitting these goals (as well as seeing a primary care physician and having your immunizations up to date—that's the "+ 2") is a key indicator of lifestyle choices that favor longevity and markers for overall health.

They do the little things that matter. Consider this personal case study. Going into a hip replacement at age 59 and then again at 64, co-author Peter was fit, did pre-therapy, and actively stuck with post-surgery physical therapy; as a result, he was able to quickly and fully recover. Peter's physical therapist noted that the usual scenario for most patients is to go into the surgery weak and ignore the post-op therapy. They blow it off, for whatever reason—perhaps thinking it's really not that important or that it hurts. This decision is the way a lot of us think about health: Why bother with the little things to change our health? Will they *really* matter that much? Yes!

Every little decision adds up, and even more as you live longer. That is what good genetic engineers do! Your lifestyle choices change the functioning of your DNA switches as surely (and in a much cheaper and easier way) than CRISPR.

Think of it this way: You build a sand castle with millions of grains of sands. Each little grain piles up into a majestic mountain of art. Same goes for your body. Every little choice builds up into the overall functioning of your body—for better or worse.

They use technology. Our greatest era of tech can also serve as an excellent support system for better health. The marketplace is full of all kinds of trackers that provide real-time and easy-to-use feedback about our health choices. You can track steps, minutes, heart rate, calories, sleep quality, and so much more. While not everyone needs tech aids or loves being tied to the taunting of our technology ("Take more steps, Frank!"), technology can provide an excellent form of motivation for many people by establishing benchmarks and goals. And it can help you in trying to reach those goals, especially when combined with the human touch of a coach. The human touch is the key to making the technology meaningful and the changes sustained.

Think about the psychological power of these measurements. Rather than being handcuffed to the judgment of our scales, we can set realistic daily goals on our devices—and make decisions every day that will give us a "win." Unlike a scale—which isn't always a true or representative measure of health—a metric that we have more control over can serve as an excellent piece of the change-making puzzle.

They leverage financial incentives. A fundamental lesson of economics is that people generally respond to incentives; it's a basic human reaction. Significant financial incentives have always been a driver of behavior change. Much of the burden of establishing those incentives comes down to how our government and industries can provide significant cash rewards for employees who are motivated to stay or get and stay healthy. But even if we look at incentives on an individual level, you and your family can improve your financial situation with better health, starting with such positives as lower medical costs, higher work productivity, a longer career, and less worry about the impacts of pandemic diseases, too.

They have a buddy or several. You need a built-in ecosystem with your own tribe—a community of people who work together and support one another in pursuit of their goals. It can come in many forms—one person, a small group of people, or a large tribe with lots of people pursuing the same goals.[9] And many people tend to experience some combination of those buddies during the evolution of a wellness journey.

Motivation theory shows that relatedness is one of the key components to long-term, intrinsic motivation. Data from EXOS (a company that trains elite athletes) shows that the factor that trumps all other factors in terms of success for special-forces fighters has nothing to do with an exercise program or protein shakes. It has to do with a specific mindset, as well as a buddy system. Having a partner (or partners) in your pursuit of behavior change is the variable that most likely predicts success.[10]

So while we will dive into the details of what the specific changes are that will best prepare you for the rebuild, there's one action you can take right now:

Find your tribe by seeking out people who share your tastes and interests.

One that understands.

One that will want to share your journey.

One that has something to give you and also needs what you have to give.

One that can build you up, prop you up, and pep you up.

And when you do, you'll be ready.

CHAPTER 13

SELF-ENGINEERING YOUR BODY

Make changes that can have exponential effects on your health and your longevity

A psychologist once told Albert that while you don't always get to choose what happens to you, you do get to choose how you deal with it. That's an important message: Control what you can control. Here are our best practices for self-engineering your body to prepare for the Great Age Reboot.

Self-Engineer Your Brain and Heart

When it comes to health strategies that can improve your body, what you do for the brain and heart are remarkably similar. That's because so much of that success hinges on a strong circulatory system and good blood flow. That's easy to imagine for the heart, since you're familiar with the idea of creating a clear vascular system through exercise and healthy eating.

It's probably harder to imagine flexing your brain. It's not like doing biceps curls to grow muscles or swimming to strengthen your heart. But even if you're not setting out to do three sets of cerebellum lifts a day, you still need to make brain self-engineering a priority when it comes to the length and quality of your life.

Our co-author Albert is still working into his 90s. While he's clever and smart and reads a lot, he thinks that one of the keys to his brain's health and longevity has to do with something else: stress management and setting priorities. "What's important is important, and the rest is baloney," he explains. (Note: We don't endorse actual bologna, as processed meat is bad for the brain and body.)

These strategies have been documented to change the way your genes are expressed and improve the systems that influence brain and heart function.

Manage stress: Research at the Cleveland Clinic has shown that people who regularly participate in stress-reducing activities dramatically decrease their perceived stress levels.[1]* This is one of the best ways to assess your ability to manage stress, since there are few medical tests that track stress levels.[2] Reducing stress helps improve markers for heart disease and brain-related problems.

MRI imaging shows that stress shrinks the hippocampus, and that atrophy is a hallmark of dementia.[3] Keep in mind that the real damage doesn't come from the stress itself, but from your

---

* One option is the Cleveland Clinic's StressFreeNow app (which is web or phone based). In it, you can choose from 12 different kinds of stress-reducing practices, such as meditation, guided imagery, deep-breathing techniques, and progressive muscle relaxation. (But for the record, Dr. Mike loves the deep-breathing techniques, putting his right index finger in his belly button and optimizing breathing patterns that way. He uses these techniques regularly, especially when some dirty-rotten SOB cuts him off in traffic. They give him a much better way to express his need to deep breathe than what he used to do.)

biological response: a cascade of hormones and chemicals during these episodes that wreak havoc on your brain and body. So the goal isn't to eliminate stress completely, but instead to improve your reaction to it.

The point of all of the techniques is that they force you to engage in a relaxing activity repeatedly, so that your focus changes and your biological systems calm down. This allows your body to recover from the processes activated by stress. This is real genetic engineering.

Move it: Exercise has all kinds of biological benefits, including decreasing stress, improving heart function, speeding up metabolism, and preventing fat storage. But perhaps the most underrated benefit is what it does for your brain:

- Numerous studies show that physical activity has a positive influence on brain function and increases the size of the hippocampus, flipping those DNA switches.[4][5][6]

- Strenuous physical activity activates genes that produce proteins released from your muscles that are small enough to get across the blood brain barrier (a sort of biological wall of tight blood vessels that prevents toxins from getting to your brain). That's important because this protein then releases another protein the brain makes called BDNF, brain-derived neurotrophic factor, which grows your hippocampus. That growth has a positive effect on brain function. Higher levels of BDNF are associated with lower risk of Alzheimer's and most forms of dementia. We go into the details of exactly what you should do for exercise in "Self-Engineering Your Fitness Plan," later in this chapter—isn't it nice to know that you can improve both body and brain in one fell swoop?

Go fish: In study after study, it's clear that one of the most potent sources of brain-friendly foods is fish—specifically, DHA and omega-3 fatty acids (and possibly omega-7).[7][8] These are most accessible in such foods as salmon and ocean trout. These friendly fats do a lot to promote good brain and heart health, including reducing damaging inflammation. Studies have also shown that regular fish eaters lose fewer brain cells than those who consume less fish, and they also show that eating fish helps arteries stay clear. (However, avoid fried fish, as well as mackerel, swordfish, tilefish, and tuna, which usually are very high in mercury.) If you're not especially fond of fish, walnuts and algal DHA supplements (see page 234) are good substitutes for DHA and omega-3 from fish and supplements for healthy fats as well. You need over 900 mg a day for your brain (based on data from a randomized study)[8] and over 1,100 mg a day for your heart based on meta-analyses [9][10]—that means about six ounces of wild salmon or 10 ounces of ocean trout every other day or its equivalent in supplements, or some combo of supplements and salmon or ocean trout.

Dial in your diet: Some research shows that a Mediterranean-style diet—or a pesco-vegetarian version that incorporates salmon, ocean trout, and a few personalized supplements—can reduce death from cardiovascular disease by up to 30 percent. Eating this way can also arrest the development of dementia by up to 60 percent.[11][12]

In a Mediterranean-influenced diet, most of your calories should come from plants or plant-based fats, like olive oil, avocados, and nuts. And, as evidenced above, a pesco-vegetarian diet, featuring salmon and ocean trout, is also best for the brain and heart in epidemiologic studies.[13] This regimen is very low in sugar, added syrups, simple carbohydrates, and saturated fat. Saturated fat (found in red meat, dairy, and egg yolks) is linked to changes in the bacteria in your intestine, which then results in the development of inflammation in over 80 percent of Americans. Inflammation can lead to heart and arterial disease, stroke, increased aging due to arthritis and the avoidance of pain by reducing movement, increased dementia, and the risk of cancer. You also should get plenty of fiber—in the form of veggies and beans, primarily—as high-fiber diets are associated with lower risks of diseases and conditions of aging associated with the arteries (from heart attacks and strokes to diabetes and inflammation).

Avoid body-busting ingredients: Fifteen straight hours of reality TV isn't the only thing that can turn your brain to marshmallow. Marshmallows can turn your brain to marshmallow—as can a few other foods:

- Avoid added sugars and syrups (found in processed foods, baked goods, and more; fruits are OK because their sugars are those found in whole food and take longer for you to process—thus they tend not to raise your blood sugar too quickly). Raising your blood sugar quickly and outside the normal range fosters biochemical processes that add plaque to your arteries, degrade your energy producing systems, add fat to your waist, foster infections, and promote inflammation everywhere in your body, leading to chronic diseases like liver and kidney failure, immune dysfunction, most cancers, and dementia.

- Avoid foods with saturated fats: It probably isn't the fat, but the proteins that come with it, that change the bacteria in your gut to cause inflammation in your brain and heart. These fats are found in red meat, egg yolks, cheese, and most other dairy; they've been linked to many health problems.

- Avoid simple carbs: Working like sugars, simple carbohydrates (found in white bread and pasta) increase your blood sugar level quickly and also trigger inflammatory responses. Whole grains and fiber are forms of carbohydrates that decrease inflammation and are good for brain and heart health (think beans, oats, fruits, and vegetables).

- Moderate alcohol is OK for your heart—no more than one and a half drinks for men and one for women daily. However, it is considered harmful for your brain. So you should make decisions about alcohol based on your personal predispositions and risk factors.

Train your brain for speed: The basic mantra here is "use it or lose it." When you're consistently working your brain, especially in places where you have to make quick decisions, you're promoting the growth of neurons, connections, and the hippocampus. Two studies found that 70- to 75-year-olds who regularly played speed-of-processing games (games in which you have to think and analyze situations quickly) for just 18 hours over a 10-year period experienced more than a 25 percent decreased risk of dementia over those 10 years, and an increase in acetylcholine (an important neurotransmitter that is key for memory recall) in key brain regions.[14][15] (We expect that playing speed games on your phone or Ping-Pong or anything that requires your brain to act fast would also be beneficial.) Now, we're not suggesting that you go out and spend your whole weekend hunkering down with Fortnite. But it is worth engaging in some games in which you process information and make decisions quickly. Because of the data supporting them, we like Double Decision and Freeze Frame from BrainHQ.

Floss your teeth daily: And prevent periodontal disease by seeing a dental professional twice a year. Oral bacteria thriving on food residue stuck between your teeth can migrate to your bloodstream. There they can fuel inflammation that damages the lining of your arteries—making it susceptible to a buildup of plaque, which stiffens and narrows the arteries and—*bang!*—heart attack, stroke, and dementia.[16]

And try this: The data clearly show that by self-engineering the switches to your genes through the actions above, you can decrease your risk of developing dementia, heart disease, and memory-related disorders. But if you're looking for an extra boost, you can add more firepower to your brain by fortifying your neurons and connections. These actions have also been shown to be beneficial:

- Drink filtered coffee (no cream or sweeteners) and enjoy blueberries. Coffee has been linked to the prevention of dementia (there is not enough data on tea or decaf coffee.) The filter eliminates diterpenes in the coffee that increase serum and LDL-cholesterol concentrations, raising the chance of cardiovascular disease and dementia.[17] Blueberries have properties that lower the risk of disease.[18]

- Eat more food early in the day and less later on. Try to eat only in a seven- or eight-hour window. Eat only when the sun is up and eat 75 percent of your calories seven or more hours before your planned bedtime.[19]

- Help regenerate your telomeres with the original Fasting Mimicking Diet (a form of intermittent fasting*) five days each month:[20] [21] Go on a low-protein, low-simple-carb diet of about 1,000 calories on day one and 750 calories for the next four days (it was mainly a tomato-corn-onion soup—32 ounces of diced tomatoes, 32 ounces of water, 12 ounces of corn niblets, 12 ounces of water, and onions and spices to taste; serve up to 17 eight-ounce portions on the 750-calorie days), and then return to a Mediterranean-style diet on day six.

- Use a sauna a few times a week. Studies demonstrate reduced dementia in more than 15 percent of those who used one four times a week for 20 minutes or more; whether this benefit is the result of stress reduction or some other property is still unknown. We believe the benefit is due to the high temperature, which releases heat shock proteins, produced by cells in response to stressful conditions. This means a hot bath or an

---

* Intermittent fasting—a catchall to describe various methods of restricted eating—does appear to have benefits for weight loss, health, and longevity. Most of the data come from studies in simple organisms and animals, where fasting has been shown to increase the life span of bacteria, yeast, worms, and mice. Studies in animals have also suggested that fasting may slow the development of some cancers and the degeneration of brain cells. Fasting can also reduce inflammation and blood pressure, as well as increase insulin sensitivity. Of course, fasting is very difficult, so scientists have been studying how to mimic its potential benefits with less extreme diets. If you're willing to give it a try, the science suggests that you may get some benefits from fasting for between 14 and 18 hours. Not eating for most of the day causes your body to burn up all its circulating glucose, as well as stored glycogen; as a result, insulin levels begin to fall. Instead of burning sugar for fuel, your body starts to rely on stored fat, which can be more easily mobilized as a result of low insulin levels. Essentially, fasting is part of what allows your body to go into a state called ketosis—in which your body uses fat for energy (as opposed to the usual sources, carbohydrates and the stored form of glycogen).

infrared sauna may have the same benefit. (Moreover, given its lower temperature, an infrared sauna doesn't make you sweat, so it can be experienced without a major change of clothes.) Heat shock proteins are released into the body by the change in temperature.)[22]

- Get six and a half to eight hours of high-quality sleep each night (see "Self-Engineer Your Immune System" below).
- Add some supplements: multivitamins and multiminerals with magnesium and calcium; vitamin D$_3$; CoQ10; a variety of healthy probiotics; baby aspirin (one in the morning and one at night with half a glass of warm water before and after)—see "Self-Engineer Your Medicine Cabinet" on page 230.

Self-Engineer Your Immune System

We cannot know for certain how quickly new medical advances will happen, what the costs will be, or how accessible these treatments and/or diagnostics will be. (You probably won't be able to go to a walk-in clinic for a kill-cancer patch in the foreseeable future.) That's why we advocate for your own self-engineering. Because one thing *is* certain: A higher functioning defense system will be your best protection against cancer and other forms of aggressive disease.

That's not to say that you can prevent or treat every serious condition by behavior alone—but you will certainly stack the odds in your favor if you do. Here's what we recommend:

Hunker down in the produce section: The absence of various micronutrients in your diet can decrease your immune function, so diversify your portfolio of leafy greens, cruciferous vegetables, berries, and citrus fruits—aim to really get a variety. This will help improve the chances that all of your micronutrients—vitamins A, B, C, D, as well as minerals like zinc and selenium—are being covered. While we do not fully understand why seasonal viruses are seasonal (and attack with much more success in the winter), it may be because in the summer the body is better protected by the increase in vitamin D_2 or D_3 produced by the greater sun's energy, or the greater moisture in the warmer air, or the more frequent consumption of fruits and vegetables with vitamin C and some micronutrients. It's also a good idea to boost your diet with half a multivitamin-multimineral supplement twice a day (morning and night) to ensure all of your bases are covered to avoid the very common zinc, magnesium, copper, and selenium deficiencies of diets in the developed world (see "Self-Engineer Your Medicine Cabinet," page 230).

Eat (the right) protein: Protein is key, since it's a building block of antibodies that are integral to your immune function. Salmon's healthy fats are good for the brain and whole body. You can also get protein from cooked beans/legumes and lean white meats, like chicken or turkey. Be aware that some sources of protein can contain large amounts of saturated fat, and the amino acids that are associated with foods with saturated fats that may promote cancer development. So stay away from red meat and processed meats. For recovery from inflammation, and cleanup of the debris after the fight between your immune system and cancer or any other invaders, you need vitamin D_2 or D_3, plus protein, plus the omega-3s and omega-7s of that salmon (or the omega-3s of walnuts or avocados), as these are hallmarks of the current research on preventing disease.

Make the cuts: For improved immune function and to help prevent cancer, it's best to limit added sugar, added syrups, and simple carbohydrates as described above. But even better, eliminate processed foods and substitute whole foods— you'll have made a key switch to improving your overall reboot.

Move, move, move: Get your motor revved. While we've talked about this above, the rationale for activity also is important for your immune system. One study that examined older adults found that physical activity was associated with a hearty production of protective T cells. Note here: Don't overexercise. Overexercising (running, biking, or otherwise training continuously for more than two hours) causes inflammation and depresses your immune system.[23] See page 204 for details and our recommendation for how much to exercise.

Don't overmedicate: Medication is one of our most important social advances; we have significantly lengthened the human life span with our ability to treat, cure, and prevent disease. That said, overmedicating can be counterproductive, as it has the potential to mess with your immune function (overriding it, in effect). Though we can't give guidelines for this because every person's case is unique, we do recommend that you discuss your medication and supplementation regimen with all of your doctors—and this also goes for any over-the-counter medications and supplements you take regularly.

If you don't allow your immune system to do its job, you're essentially taking away its ability to "practice." And when it's out of practice, it can't perform when it really needs to. So, while we're not saying that you should skip the doctor and leave a sinus infection untreated, we are saying that you should think twice about popping pain-relief medication like candy. Ditto acid blockers for heartburn: Your own stomach acid offers a great defense in killing invaders; taking acid blockers negates this part of your defense system.

Get your vaccines: Stay up to date, and get an annual flu shot. The flu increases overall inflammation, and research shows that getting an annual flu shot for 10 years, from ages 50 to 60, decreases heart attacks and strokes by 50 percent and death in this age group by 25 percent, probably by decreasing the inflammation that accompanies the flu, and the plaque breakage that inflammation causes.[24] [25] The vaccine for COVID-19 prevention must be added to prevent heart attacks, strokes, memory loss, and kidney disease that may result from COVID-19 inflammation. Taking a multivitamin for several weeks and getting great sleep for several days prior to a flu shot boosts the flu shot's success in protecting you from the influenza viruses.[26] [27]

Take time for YOU: One of the major threats to your immune system is chronic stress; the cascade of hormonal responses it causes weakens your immune function over time. Chronic stress can lead to a buildup of cytokines, which, while fighting infection, can also hurt your own cells in the process. And yet, in some circles, "self-care" is an eight-letter four-letter word. People pooh-pooh the idea of self-care because, they say, either a) they don't have time or b) they're too tough (*"I don't need no stinking self-care"*). And we get it; it's our nature to put others before ourselves. But as the Cleveland Clinic's great gynecologist Linda Bradley says, "You can't pour from an empty cup!!!"

Think of it this way: If you don't take time to care for yourself, you won't be around long enough to be with the people you really want to help and be with anyway. While there's no such thing as total stress relief (after all, stress is simply a byproduct of living a fulfilling and challenging life), there are ways to self-engineer the effects that negative and chronic stress can have on your body.

Here are some of the top things you can do to help squash stress (speaking of which, Dr. Mike was a top squash player back in the day, and believes friendships formed from sports and games are key to relationship building, which in turn fosters stress relief!):

Meditation: Research has shown that meditation can help improve telomere length (telomeres are at the end of DNA and shorter ones are associated with aging), and thus improve overall health and decrease stress response. Even just a few minutes of meditation a day can be helpful, and there are a number of apps and online videos that can help you get started.

Deep breathing: Deep breathing engages the relaxation response. Really think about pulling those breaths from your belly and diaphragm.

Better emotional connections: Social support is key for helping to reduce the negative effects of stress. In fact, social contact with at least six different people a month has long been associated with a number of positive outcomes: Studies show that blood markers for immune response are different between lonely people and those who are social. And kindness to others also generates better immune functioning. No matter what age or stage you're in, you need to find a tribe (if you don't have one) or regularly engage with yours (if you do).[28]

Quality and quantity of sleep: This is probably one of our population's greatest self-engineering issues. Poor sleep is associated with decreased immune function and premature aging from infectious processes. That means you need to not only get enough sleep (at least 6.5 hours every night), but also make sure it's quality sleep. Good sleep hygiene (no screens in the bedroom, no eating for at least three hours before sleep, only red-wavelength lights in bathrooms, etc.) is crucial to making sure you get your rest. Try lying on your back with a pillow under your knees as a way of improving sleep and decreasing inflammation at night (however, if you snore or have sleep apnea, you should not lie on your back when you sleep, unless you use CPAP). Sleeping more than 6.5 hours a night before every immunization plus a multivitamin for at least 3 weeks prior has been shown to importantly increase the success rate of every vaccine where such has been tested.

Self-Engineer Your Fitness Plan

It's easy for us to say, "Hey, you should get off the couch and exercise," but when you understand a bit more of why activity works, it can be a helpful psychological tool to use when trying to drum up the motivation to get going. Activity is one of the best things you can do for your heart, your brain, and your musculoskeletal system. (One note: Anyone with a history or family history of heart disease should consult medical professionals before starting an exercise plan that is more strenuous than what you have done in the past two weeks.)

Some of the benefits:
- A study by London researchers found that during exercise, the cartilage in your joints gets squished. This actually prevents the degradation of cartilage (as the movement suppresses the action of inflammatory molecules associated with osteoarthritis).[29]
- Studies show that being sedentary is associated with a

higher risk of a number of problems, including cardio-vascular disease.[30]

- Exercise can reverse heart damage for people who have been sedentary. Research has shown that this happens because physical activity helps improve the heart's elasticity and function.[31]
- Maintaining and adding a little muscle mass helps boost your metabolism, because muscle is metaboli-cally expensive. You burn more calories just by having muscle instead of fat. That is a virtuous cycle.
- Research has shown that strength training can signifi-cantly reduce the symptoms associated with depres-sion, including anxiety, apathy, low mood, and sadness.[32]
- Exercise helps you maintain body mass without gaining fat. A study in the journal *Clinical Interventions in Aging* found that losing mass (and replacing it with fat) with age can be associated with memory problems such as dementia.[33]

So where to start? Well, first, any exercise is better than no exercise, but think of 60 minutes a day of purposeful move-ment (a few minutes every half hour you're awake) as an excel-lent baseline to commit to. We would also like you to think about making sure that you cover all of your bases, so we rec-ommend varying your routine for the most powerful effects.

Our recommendations include:
- Walking 10,000 steps a day (or the equivalent—approxi-mately one minute of activity equals 100 steps). You could be on a bike or elliptical machine, swimming, carrying

groceries, gardening—they all count. Every day, no excuses.

- Some form of resistance training two or three days a week (doing this and counting repetitions of an exercise can be a form of meditation, as it clears your mind). See pages 207–208 for more on the specifics, and make sure you also strengthen your core for the long run and to avoid back pain in the meantime.

- Cardiovascular exercise (running, walking briskly, swimming, cycling) with enough intensity to increase your heart rate three times a week for 20 minutes to at least 80 percent of your age-adjusted maximum heart rate (approximately 220 minus your age for both men and women). One study shows that going beyond the recommended maximum heart rate with high-intensity interval training—putting out maximum effort for 20 seconds of every two minutes of that 20 minutes more than three times a week and getting to more than 80 percent of your age-adjusted maximum heart rate— decreases disability, dementia, and death. A study in the British journal *Sports Medicine* found that you can reduce your risk of all-cause mortality by 24 percent if you increase your walking pace to a brisk one (the study looked at walkers who reached 4.3 miles per hour). Or you can integrate interval training—going for one minute hard and then two minutes at a moderate pace (alternating for about 20 minutes). You can do this with running, biking, swimming, even walking. (While there is substantial data proving that this kind of high-intensity interval training [HIIT] improves fitness, only that one study has so far shown that it increases length of life.)[34]

- About 40 jumps in place a day. This is an important activity for increasing lymphatic flow, as well as for increasing bone density and spinal disk health. Just as weightlifting increases muscle strength by inflicting small injuries to your muscles so they become stronger, jumping inflicts small injuries to your bone and disks— and what doesn't break you makes you younger.[35] [36]

Need some help getting started with a workout? Taking a brisk walk is a perfectly great place to start. But it's also important to work your muscles in different ways, too. The following simple, 30-minute workout will help get you started. You can adapt it to make it harder or easier, depending on your fitness level and how you progress.

Set a digital timer for 30 minutes. Every time a minute hits (at :00), perform one exercise for the prescribed amount of time or repetitions. Then do the next exercise at the next minute mark. Do fewer reps or for a shorter time if you need to, or add reps or time if you need more of a challenge. Do this three times a week.

10 exercises: Do one after the other, and then repeat the circuit two more times to complete the 30-minute quota

1. March in place (with high knees) at a "walking" speed for 20 seconds.
2. Squat in place for 10 repetitions (keep your thighs parallel to the ground when you lower yourself).
3. Do push-ups on your knees or toes for five repetitions. If that's too hard, start by doing them standing up and pushing against a wall.

4. Jump in place for 20 seconds.

5. Plank for 15 seconds. Put yourself in the "up" part of a pushup position and hold it. Keep your back flat and your butt down.

6. March in place for 20 seconds, slightly faster than the first time you did it.

7. Squat in place, but slowly—taking three full seconds to lower yourself and three full seconds to stand. Do squats for 30 seconds.

8. "Bear crawl." On your hands and toes, crawl around the room for 20 seconds.

9. "Shadow box" for 45 seconds. With your knees slightly bent, punch the air in a boxing motion, alternating punches between right and left arms.

10. Touch your toes and hold the stretch for the entire minute.

Self-Engineer Against Accidents and Mistakes ("Unforced Errors")

You can have the best body in the world, but if your hobby is skateboarding off cliffs, your risk of accidentally dying increases. These kinds of variables are what we call unforced errors. In tennis, those are the shots that you should make but miss, through nothing that your opponent did to make the play difficult. Millions struggle by making avoidable mistakes. These are the most common:

#1 Not Getting Preventive Care: Early detection of any health issue is one of the major keys to treating it before it ages you too early. Remember, bad cells re-create themselves. Your body is a resilient thing of beauty, but the further down a bad path you are, the harder it is to get back to where you need to be. Unfortunately, many people ignore annual physical exams and other diagnostics. Make these your regular appointments:

- Physical exam: annually, including blood and other tests to help you minimize heart disease, stroke, and orthopedic, metabolic, and dementia risks.
- Colonoscopy: every three to 10 years after the age of 45 depending on findings for prior colonoscopies and your risk factors (some with unique risk factors, such as African Americans at age 40, may need one earlier).
- Gynecological and urologic exams: yearly.
- Mammograms in women and men with gynecomastia: every one to two years from age 30 till your RealAge is over 84.
- Others: eyes, ears, smell, one leg standing, grip strength, and bone density tests every two years after age 50.

Longevity bonus: A thin-slice whole-body MRI to detect early cancer has been advocated by some longevity specialists at age 60 and every five years thereafter, but please discuss with your doctor the "incidentomas" that are often discovered. These are tumors that are incidentally discovered, and you are told need to be "investigated with a biopsy or surgery." Many of these can remain undisturbed the rest of your life without harming you. The risk in discovering them is in the anxiety they cause if nothing is done about them, as well as the risks of surgery if you do something about them. You should discuss what you will do for them *before* undergoing this MRI. The procedure has no doubt saved some lives, but it has also caused much anxiety and needless surgical removal of tumors.

The Link Between Mammograms and Heart Disease

Digital mammograms reveal more than your risk for breast cancer. They can spot calcium deposits in your breasts' blood vessels. Research estimates that around 10 percent of women in their 40s have what's called breast arterial calcification (BAC), and by the time they're in their 80s, around 50 percent of women do. Preliminary studies indicate that BAC is a sign you are at an increased risk for heart attack, stroke, and heart failure.[37] So, when you get your mammogram, ask specifically if you have BAC. If you do, schedule an appointment with a cardiologist to assess your risk. Changing your diet, taking a statin, lowering your blood pressure, getting more physical activity—these changes can reduce your risk for heart attack and stroke by 50 percent or more.

#2 Ignoring the Doctor's Advice: Research shows that less than a quarter of people who are prescribed cardiac rehab after a cardiovascular incident or procedure actually go.[38] How about physical therapy exercises after an accident or injury? Taking your medication for the entire timeline? There's a reason doctors and physiotherapists prescribe activities, medication, and other interventions. So just because you "feel just fine now" doesn't mean you should shortcut the R_x from your medical professionals. We're not saying that failure to do so is always intentional. A 2018 survey published in the *Journal of the American Medical Association* found that more than a third of patients don't tell their doctors if they disagree with or don't understand treatment recommendations.[39] Not speaking up may come from embarrassment or fear of looking like you don't know something. But if you don't ask questions, the thing that's ultimately hurt isn't your ego; it's your whole body.

#3 Not Getting a Second Opinion: Every doctor and health professional travels at a different speed. Some are up on their research, some aren't. Health and medicine are complicated—especially as you get into serious stuff—so you need to seek out multiple opinions. One study found that more than 30 percent of people over the age of 30 who were diagnosed with type 2 diabetes actually had type 1.[40] And 30 percent of biopsies diagnosed by pathologists as breast cancer weren't actually malignant. Second opinions (which should be sought for any decision or medical treatment that will last longer than three days, in our opinion) exist not to create conflict, but to create alternative approaches—and to reinforce the first opinion or diagnosis.[41] In the age of telemedicine, these are easier and easier to do—and doctors welcome them. In ideal cases, the two doctors (or three if you like) can actually discuss the pluses and minuses of their approaches and come to a consensus. So it may not always be a "one is right, and one is wrong" scenario, but an opportunity to get a team discussing the best approaches to your situation.

#4 Ignoring What Your Body Is Telling You: Your body is the greatest feedback mechanism ever built. It wants to give you feedback all the time. Pain, for instance, tells you to take your hand out of the crocodile's mouth. Breathing heavily after walking up the stairs tells you that your heart and/or lungs aren't working as efficiently as they used to. Being unable to buckle your belt tells you that maybe you've had #toomanytacos. But what good is feedback if you ignore it? None. So you have to be open to your body's messages not just in dire circumstances but every day. Consider these examples:

- *High blood pressure* is an indicator and cause of every-thing from heart problems to cognitive issues—it's one of the biggest warning signs the body has (and it's espe-cially vital because high BP usually has no outward symptoms that you can feel). This also underscores the importance of taking your BP regularly (it's a no-brainer with the availability of home and in-store monitors). Try to, no DO, keep it under 125 systolic and 85 diastolic.

- *Snoring* does more than just cause middle-of-the-night pillow attacks between spouses. Snoring is associated with heart problems, hypertension, depression, type 2 diabetes, sleep apnea, and more. Ignoring it—without knowing what may be causing it—is just allowing a health problem to fester and put you at higher risk of complications.

#5 Falling for Fraud: You obviously want to avoid financial fraud, someone stealing your hard-earned savings. Remem-ber: If it seems too good to be true, it most certainly is. Then there is the challenge of medical fraud. This is a tricky one—and it's going to get even trickier as more advances develop and more imposters emerge. How do you know what's helpful and what's snake oil? How do you know what methods are backed by science or ahead of the science? How do you know who to trust? This underscores the need for having a good team in place, so you can triangulate opinions and perspectives, as well as do your own research. The devel-opments below, we suspect, will be some of the warning-zone arenas that will be rife with dangerous or misleading infor-mation, services, and/or products.

- *Stem cells:* Stem cells and growth factors from specific exosomes are likely to be one of our major break-throughs—and being able to use their strength for cellular healing and rejuvenation most probably will be part of the Great Age Reboot. However, many companies now are claiming to do more in this arena than they actually can (it's currently a $3 billion industry in the United States, largely fraudulent). In the United States, except under specific clinical trials approved by the FDA (only two were approved as of mid-2020), it is illegal to perform stem cell therapies. That has driven the practice offshore, where it is not as well regulated.

- *Supplements:* While many supplements do have science behind them, others are nothing more than wallet biopsies. One prime example: Many protein supplements are touted to help skin but have no quality science to support their use as oral supplements. Same with certain well-advertised-on-TV brain supplements to improve memory—they did so exactly as well as placebos on repeat testing. Take the same test twice and tests show you are likely to improve just as much with or without that supplement. We discuss in the next chapter which supplements have enough science to review with your doctor.

- *Generic contamination:* As reported in Katherine Eban's wonderful book *Bottle of Lies*, medications can be contaminated due to mass production, or can be fraudulently produced to give you 10 percent or 30 percent of what's on the label.[42] Our solution: Buy only from a pharmacy that verifies that what's on the label is in the bottle. Valisure, for example, is a start-up pharmacy that has grown at an incredible rate; it offers a specific examination to confirm that the right amount of each ingredient is present in each batch of pills it receives from drug manufacturers or wholesalers (we have no vested interest in this company). If drug contamination and fraudulent fulfillment continue (and they have been going on for more than 10 years), we expect Walmart and other big-box pharmacies, as well as academic centers like the Cleveland Clinic, to begin using verification methods similar to Valisure's for their medications.

CHAPTER 14

SELF-ENGINEERING YOUR LIFE

New ways to think about everything from your retirement to your relationships

There's more to building a better and stronger body than just making sure the mechanics of your physical self are in good working order. There's a strong case to be made that the financial, social, and relational areas of your life are equally crucial to your overall well-being.

Self-Engineer Your Wealth

Managing your money can feel like trying to cross the Pacific on a paddleboard, especially in times of turbulent markets. It's a lot of work, sometimes it hurts, and you can feel like you're going nowhere or even backward. This is why having a team around you is helpful, since it can help you avoid money mistakes that many people make. The big ones include:

Not saving enough: Saving early and saving enough to ensure financial stability for the Great Age Reboot is your number-one financial priority. Rather than forcing yourself to take money out of your paycheck and deposit it into a savings or retirement account, automate the action so it's tucked away *before* you even see it.

Where should you invest your money? The best option is a diversified market index fund in a retirement account. Automate it, forget about it, and go about life. One note: Most people who can benefit from the tax advantages of retirement savings tax often don't put aside enough. So stretch yourself—and, if you can, put most of every raise into that account—and you will reap the benefits down the road. If your company rewards you with reduced premiums for health insurance when you achieve healthy biomarkers, put that money into a health savings account (or in a Roth IRA if no HSA is available) and convert the HSA to a retirement account after age 65.

Waiting too long: As with exercise, you can't keep putting it off. Start—or restart—now. Saying you'll do it tomorrow adds up to a whole lot of tomorrows over the course of a year or years.

Getting emotional: You want to avoid knee-jerk reactions (to the market, to family situations, etc.). Your best financial decisions don't come in the heat of the moment; they come when things have calmed down. When it comes to money, the executive part of your brain needs to override the reptilian part. Save your emotion for vacation planning, anniversary gifts, and when your team wins or loses—not for money decisions.

Thinking your home is a can't-lose investment: While real estate (like most real assets) tends to improve in value, that's not always the case. There are many variables (values in the neighborhood, overall economic climate, and more), so you can't bank on the fact that your home will always appreciate in value.

Banking on lenders: Almost always, debt creates more problems than it solves. And while it's tempting not to, living within your means will help ensure financial security.

Being too active: Buy, sell, trade—you think you can outsmart the market with lots of transactions. The better play is the patient—and yes, unexciting—one. There are risks and fees associated with a lot of movement, so establishing your portfolio with a good asset allocation and then just waiting over the long haul will most likely pay the biggest dividends.

Not doing regular checkups: Just like you should have a physical every year, you should also take a stethoscope to your portfolio. It's smart to see what you have, how it's trending, and to talk with your financial advisers about whether or not you should tinker with it. You don't need to make hasty decisions, but you should assess regularly and make well-informed ones. And never buy "because it's up" or sell "because it's down." The horse is out of the barn by then.

Self-Engineer Your Retirement

If you're old enough to remember a generation or two ago, you probably have a notion of how retirement looked. You'd have had one or two employers and it was more than likely that you'd done basically the same thing for your entire career—perhaps getting promoted, perhaps doing the same task day in and day out. At about age 65, you'd hang it up and spend the rest of your years living a simple life on whatever you had saved for your retirement and/or whatever pension your employer provided.

Fast-forward to today's workers. They change jobs more frequently and maybe even reinvent themselves, depending on their skill set. Indeed, they might never hold a steady job, instead weaving together a variety of income sources to live a more flexible life. But they still have that same old sweet spot—62 to 70—as their desired age for retirement and living the "good life" that their savings will allow.

So what happens in the Great Age Reboot? What happens when some 47 million people will be over the age of 90—and perhaps 25 to 40 percent of them will still be part of the workforce, because they'll be more like the 55- to 60-year-olds of today, and 40-year-olds of the 1960–80s, still healthy, still vital, still able to contribute meaningfully?

Your career may no longer be simple or traditional. It may be *many* careers. We predict that there will be a mass sense of reinvention when it comes to working. Our work lives won't just span the 40 or so years they do now, but will go on for perhaps 60 or 70 years, so people may want several meaningful careers.

By 2050, in a rebooted world, we predict the typical retirement age will be much closer to 80 than today's 65, and retirement benefits will generally not kick in until age 75. Those in retirement will have greater health and "be" younger than any previous retirement cohort. While they may not have the savings to live out their fantasy retirement, they will be better prepared for it than any other cohort in history. They will have benefited from generous inheritances and many more years of defined contribution savings, resulting in wealth levels and retirement incomes that were unimaginable in the past.

A big unanswered question is what will people do with their additional monetary resources and years. We suspect that as bodies feel and behave younger, the demand to look commensurately younger will skyrocket. (After all, if I feel this good, I will want to look this good as well!) Expect more and more effective cosmetic surgery and treatments to become the norm, and perhaps even genetically rebooted skin—without wrinkles! (See "Self-Engineer Your Appearance" on page 244 for more on keeping your skin looking younger.)

The effect of increased longevity is that you will earn more money than any generation before—and thus have even more to use as discretionary spending. The collective effect on the country's economics will be substantial.

Retirement also brings up some deeper questions, ones that have an effect on you and your health.

First, what do you want to do with your life? What will you be happy doing? What are your contributions to society? What gives you a sense of greater purpose?

These questions become even more important in terms of careers (and career shifting) before your main earning time is up. All kinds of jobs will exist in 2050 that we have never dreamed of today. *Why yes, Frank, we are interested in travel agents who specialize in Neptune!* As technology and society change, so do the support structures—which puts a greater emphasis on an individual's ability to adapt and to work within new frameworks.

The bottom line, when it comes to rebooted retirement, is that it's not just about a new "length of service." It's also a mindset shift, in which you're only partially defined by what you do. Other criteria include how well you adapt to a variety of careers—ones that will hopefully give you a sense of purpose, satisfaction, and optimism. Some things to consider when it comes to a new approach to retirement:

- Zero in on the aspects of your work that you love and physically can do and focus on those.
- Examine educational opportunities to develop skills in new areas that will allow you to keep pursuing your passions.
- Assuming you're financially stable, consider a second (or third or fourth) career in new areas in which you're motivated by passion, rather than money.

Self-Engineer Your Relationships

When you give advice or forecast the future, it's easy to get bogged down in science and stats: organ transplants, compound interest, what have you. And while there's a lot to discuss about progress, about process, about the playbook kind of X's and O's, we can't describe the Great Age Reboot without a nod to the hugs-and-kisses X's and O's. The Beatles were on to something when they said, "All you need is love." That's because they go hand in hand—your body and your mind, science and soul, your anatomical heart and your metaphorical heart.

As the world reboots, little of it matters without a larger consideration of things that are meaningful to you: who you are and what you do with your life. (As columnist and author David Brooks once noted, Are you living your eulogy or your résumé?)[1]

One thing is certain: The Great Age Reboot will change the dynamics of your family structure (including nonbiological family) and the nature of the working world in a way we have never seen before. And while this will require a go-with-the-flow attitude as you age, it helps to think about what's ahead.

Today, when it comes to family trees, we tend to think of three living generations: children, parents, and grandparents.

Of course, that formula varies; because of early deaths, some may not have grandparents while others may have great-grandparents. We tend to forget that earlier generations rarely knew their grandparents at all.

Over time, our family trees have grown more complicated as divorce rates soar and birth rates fall. Oftentimes, it's not about just one family unit, but several layers of extended and blended families that branch out in different directions. If you do not have children, you may have a loving, nonbiological family.

Now, take our existing structure and add some 40 years to the average life span. What happens? You have perhaps five generations instead of three as the typical unit: children, parents, grandparents, great-grandparents, great-great-grandparents, and nonbiological family. Add in the fact that people will still have life bumps and changes, divorce will still happen, and blended families will grow.

Families will become tribes rather than small units.

Most of all, enhanced longevity underscores the importance of strong relationships—romantic, familial, and platonic—as they are a major source of optimum health. Keeping connected as we age is critical, especially for the very old (relationships keep us in the present, not the past). When we're younger, relationships help us personalize empathy.

Replenishing friends and love connections is essential throughout life, whether it's when you attend a new school as a seven-year-old or when you retire. Friends and family die, move, and shift their priorities. You must replace them or become isolated by attrition—and this takes work. (One of the worst things about the COVID-19 shutdown was that it eroded this key health factor because of the isolation that came with it, which both increased stress and may have contributed to economic worries.)

Grandchildren are a good place to start, but they're often far away or uninterested. So that means it's about creating your preferred "family." And it may not be by bloodline. Remember that your spouse is not blood. A "love family" may include blood relatives, but why be so limited? "Love family" can outlast blood, but it takes openness and love and effort.

Needless to say, the quality (and existence) of your relationships has a significant effect on your health. Consider this research:

- Social isolation—the absence of family, which is all too common in the aging population—increases the effects of stress, as well as the risk of death and serious disease. This is especially important to recognize, since nearly 43 percent of people say they're lonely at any given time.
- Married people who rated their marriages as "very happy" or "pretty happy" had 20 percent lower odds of dying over any 10-year period than people who didn't report happiness in their marriages. (Men seem to benefit more by being married: A happy heterosexual marriage makes a man about three years younger and a woman about two years younger at age 55. An unhappy marriage makes a man no older but a woman three years older.)
- Older adults with larger social networks are better at staying ahead of the game when it comes to self-engineering and making lifestyle choices for optimal health. Those who weren't as socially engaged were

33 percent more likely to miss preventive services or screenings and experienced much higher levels of stress, as well as stress-associated aging and dementia. Social connections are the key to mitigating stress's adverse effects on your body and brain functions.

The key to loving relationships, research has found, is what's called "emotional responsiveness." This is just what it sounds like: being there for the people around you, not physically, but in an emotionally engaged way. This applies not just to romantic relationships, but to friendships as well.

Self-Engineer Your Sex Life

It's no secret that as we age, sexual function can decrease, for a variety of reasons. Some are mechanical (translation: When blood flow is weakened from arterial aging, blood can't reach the sexual organs). Some are psychological (emotions are highly tied to arousal). And some are simply logistical (stressful days can mean that the bed looks a lot better for sleeping than it does for bebopping).

That said, that doesn't mean you should write off sexual dysfunction as an inevitable part of aging, since a healthy sex life in a healthy relationship has many (besides the obvious) advantages.

Physically, the most common problem for men is erectile dysfunction—the inability to get or maintain an erection. Medications can help, but doing things that improve blood flow (physical activity, eating well) can also improve circulation to the area. For women, because of hormonal changes that happen after menopause, lack of lubrication and arousal are common, underscoring the importance of not only blood flow, but also intimacy and understanding that the bodies of today are not the bodies of yesterday (translation: spending more time on foreplay). The most important variable for still having sex at age 75 (other than having a partner): your degree of inflammation (as detected by a blood test for hsCRP) for subjects aged 58.[2] And as we've learned, to a large degree, you can genetically and epigenetically engineer your inflammation level to be lower. That's one reason we recommend getting that blood test with your yearly LDL checkup. Tests to help you gauge inflammation include a full alphabet: hsCRP, MPO, OxLDL, ApoB, TMAO, IL-6, FP-Iso, ADMA, and others.

In addition, many health problems, including pain, depression, heart disease, and the medications used to treat them—another reason for that second opinion—can come with a side effect of sexual dysfunction. And that reinforces one of our main points: Taking care of yourself holistically has a positive effect on all aspects of your life.

Self-Engineer Your Social Life

Being socially engaged is one of the most important things you can do for your mind, for your health, for your life. It's not always easy to do—especially if your tendency is to hole up on your couch, search Netflix, and retreat when the going gets tough. We can't recommend a one-size-fits-all approach. What works for one may be hellish for another, so we asked some folks in our inner circle for some ideas—partly to give you some ideas, but mostly to inspire you to make sure this is one of your priorities as you age:

"I joined a Tai Chi group (good for my health and includes others looking to connect socially), have phone dates to maintain friendships (no texting) with friends that live in other places, and commit to 'birthday dates' with three friends even if scheduling means doing it weeks after the actual birthday." —Jill, 63

"We organize lunches, dinners, rounds of golf, reunions and mini reunions, ski trips, and golf trips." —Warren, 75

"I play tennis and platform tennis, so we play socially and on competitive teams. Through this route I have connected with a large network of couples as well as ladies—in addition to playing tennis we go out to the movies, out to dinner, have card parties, and have even gone on vacation together. I am actively involved with my daughter's youth sports, I am the parent representative and on the school athletic boosters. I have made friends this way, parents who will go out before or after games and volunteer with our teenagers. My husband and daughter and I have a group chat where we communicate all day long with everything from dinner plans to daily successes to jokes/memes. We also volunteer as a family at our church. My nieces and nephews are in their 20s and communicate on Snapchat. They are all out of town and it is very fun and easy to send one another snaps. Even my nephew, who is in Afghanistan, is able to Snapchat with me frequently. I LOVE this." —Holli, 50

"A fun way I stay connected to friends and family is an app called Marco Polo. It's a video message app. I have a group video chat going each day with three of my best friends from childhood, one with my mom and sister-in-law, and another with friends from my days living in New York. The messages not only update me on what everyone is up to, but most importantly, keep me laughing each day." —Ann, 69

"We stay in touch with family using FaceTime. Our kids often show their grandparents around the house, make silly faces, and they always make sure our guinea pig, Shaggy, gets to squeak hello too." —Erica, 41

"Forty-five years ago, six couples benefited a high school auction by buying a donated ski weekend at a Vermont chalet. It was just the first of 20 subsequent trips we took together over the years to places as far-flung as Istanbul. Group shopping, assigned tasks for dinner cooking and cleanup, assigned pre-reads for discussion, long walks, and cemented friendships uniquely bonded these devoted 12 in matchless moments of joy, humor, and memory. Seven of us have since died, but the five remaining, despite living far apart, are still umbilically close and connected." —Jack, 72

"Calling my mom and dad makes them so happy or even just sending a greeting card to say I love you. It's critically important to have these human connections." —Ivy, 54

"These days, I spend a lot of time traveling. I have found that people my age (who are not 'connected' to music or video games, which are inherently solitary activities) who travel are quite open to starting or engaging in conversation at airports or on planes. Sometimes, it starts as idle chatter about the weather, or a flight delay, or what someone is reading. It often turns to more substantive conversation, the exchange of business cards, and sometimes, a friendship or partnership. I met my current business partner at baggage claim in Akron, Ohio, years ago when we both realized from simultaneous conversations we were having that we had a common business interest." —Jeff, 61

"I meet up once a year in a new city with several other friends from my time as a Navy wife. There are four of us and we always have a blast just catching up and seeing the sights of whatever city we happen to choose. This year it will be Nashville." —Tonia, 57

"Google empowers us to be experts at just about anything. We will be at dinner and a subject comes up I know nothing about. No more concerns that I look uninformed or cannot participate in the conversation, I just Google—it's great for impressing old friends and making new ones." —Mary, 62

"A few years ago, my husband and I moved from an area where we had lived for 48 years to be closer to our family. We knew we were leaving behind our home of 42 years but, more importantly, our network of friends. One of our first priorities was to establish a new network of friends. This takes time and effort and openness. It is trite but true, you need to be a friend to make friends. Making friends is a reason for getting up in the morning, for sharing activities like book groups and mah-jongg groups. Friends have included us in family holiday meals, allowing us not to feel alone. All of this means there must be reciprocity. Friends provide phone calls, meals, visits during times of surgery or illness or loss. They make us feel cared about and not alone. Yes, this all takes time. But without social contacts, there is loneliness and too much concern about one-self." —Marsha, 78

"A passion of mine is volunteering in my community. It can be serving the homeless children, reading to shut-ins, or escorting the elderly to medical appointments or going for walks out-doors. I've made a great circle of like-minded friends who also enjoy supporting others in need. Volunteering not only helps those we serve but gives those of us in the support roles a great sense of gratitude. I also established years ago with my friends a 'no gift-giving' policy for birthdays and Christmas. Instead, I asked those who insisted in gifting me to donate several hours of their time in community service. It's amazing the number of folks who initially hesitated and now have adopted the same policy. I've made a great circle of friends with this practice. Paying it forward . . . " —Donna, 67

"My high school and college friends make a very concerted effort to get together each year in a different part of the country. We may golf, fish, or spend a couple days exploring a city and grabbing great food. It's a terrific time filled with bragging about our families and reliving old memories!" —Wael, 50

"I use every opportunity to communicate with my friends and family. Anytime I am sitting in the back of a cab, airports, or trains I use the time to send a note to my closest friends and family. I speak with my children and my mother every day. With my sister several times a week. Frequency of communication is important, much more so than duration. These techniques have helped me to stay in touch with my family and friends in Croatia even though I left it 30 years ago." —Tom, 56

"Making friends takes time; keeping friends takes time. For most of my life, from being a farm kid, through college and grad school, while running several businesses and editing six texts, I worked 50 to 70 hours a week. I acquired lots of things, aka 'toys.' During this time, my brothers (my best friends who live within 20 minutes of me), who were always employed full time, enjoyed their lives with their friends. Lots of parties, camping, snowmobiling, boating, hunting, socializing . . . creating fun with other people. As I neared retirement, and even more so after retirement, I had more time. When I would call my brothers to do something, usually involving some 'toy' or other, they were off with their friends appreciating something else. They rarely had time for me then, and they don't really have time now because they always have 'something going on.' Although we really have fun when we get together, they have tons of friends, while I have 'things.' I've come to realize that friendships need time to be nurtured. They take some effort. Friendships don't just happen and exist without attention. They must be cultivated with care and they especially need the fertilizer of 'time.' I've experienced another epiphany too: Great friendships and social networks can occur even later in life if they are deemed to be a priority.

"It's necessary that you give of yourself to grow friends . . . give some time. It takes willingness to share yourself, your feelings, your caring, the readiness to listen. It involves some risk . . . but the happiest memories don't seem to be about acquiring the 'toys.' It's the enduring friendships.

"A few friends and I mostly use email to keep in touch. Email allows for daily (in some cases, just occasional) conversational, serious, or funny connections with another human being who is special in my life. It allows me to feel not only acknowledged but this connectedness [I feel] is as important to the other person as it is to me. There are three distinct groups of friends—small social networks—that I email almost daily. They are each different. One is comprised of retired colleagues, another of veterans, and there is also a group of family members. My children make up a fourth group. Living in a time when all of our lives are so filled and so busy, it's enjoyable to take a few minutes each day to tune into email and savor this continuation of a relationship. Since it's unobtrusive, we can check in at leisure when we have a few minutes—it's a rewarding experience and makes 'receiving that letter' so much more readily available!" —Jack, 72

Self-Engineer Your Medicine Cabinet

In an ideal world, the food you eat would provide you all the vitamins, minerals, and micro- and macronutrients needed to power your body. But research shows that when it comes to the recommended daily values (DV) or recommended daily intake (RDI) of nutrients, 99.9 percent of us fail to take in 100 percent of what's recommended and only 7 percent get more than 20 percent of the daily value of all vitamins and minerals. Here are the vitamins, minerals, supplements, and medications shown to reduce aging and improve longevity that we would recommend you talk to your doc about, and a few others antiaging researchers take themselves due to great animal data (but not yet proven in us humans):

Vitamin D$_3$

Why you should take it: Between 42 and 82 percent of the population is vitamin D deficient. This almost certainly shortens longevity.[3] Research shows a blood level of 35 ng/ml or higher of D$_3$ has an array of benefits: It protects against cancer, protects arteries from the effects of aging, *reverses* diabetes, protects against erectile dysfunction—even reduces all-cause mortality.[4] While the data are pretty clear that a D$_3$ level of 35 keeps you able to make your body function younger than a level of 10 or 20, we do not know that D$_3$ levels of 50 or 80 are necessarily better than 35. And in truth, we do not know that supplementing to levels over 35 reduces the diseases and conditions associated with levels less than 35. But we postulate it does, and we know 35 is better than 15.

What to be cautious about: So get a blood test annually to find out what level of D$_3$ supplementation you need to boost your level to at least 35 (though we prefer to shoot for a level of 50 to 80 ng/ml). Toxicity rarely appears till levels exceed 107 ng/ml.[5]

How much to take: Until you know the results of that blood test start taking 1,000 IU daily, but personalize your dosage. You need more the older you are, as you do not absorb or make D$_3$ as well as you gain years.

Multivitamin/multimineral

Why you should take it: Most of us are missing some portion of the essential vitamins and minerals. And there are good data—especially when it comes to the effects on longevity. Research reveals that taking a multivitamin for more than 10 years decreases cancer rates (and by more than 8 percent for non-prostate cancers in men over 65).[6][7] Half a multi twice a day keeps your heart younger and pumping stronger, as it decreases overt cardiovascular disease by over 25 percent (and probably disease that is covert but slows you down), as shown in the 20-year follow-up of the Health Professionals study.[8]

What to be cautious about: Do not take extra vitamins like those added to bottled water or food unless monitored by your doctor, as more can do more harm than good. For example, some excess B vitamins from supplements are associated with increased breast cancer or premature death.[9] [10]

How much to take: Split a multi; take half in the morning, half at night (this will keep nutrient blood levels closer to constant). Stick with a multi with nutrient doses that are close to their daily value or RDI (since super-spiking one nutrient with extra amounts can throw off the working relationship between nutrients and do more harm than good).

Calcium citrate and magnesium

Why you should take it: Calcium keeps you functioning as if you are younger in many ways, including building bone strength. Adequate calcium intake is essential for healthy bones and teeth, for muscles to function, and for nerves to carry messages. Calcium is also used to help release hormones and enzymes that keep your body going. Generally, folks get about half the daily calcium they need (~1,200 mg) from diet, so take a 600 mg daily supplement that has 300 mg of magnesium, which helps counteract the constipation complication associated with calcium. Calcium also helps prevent insomnia, helps regulate muscle and nerve function, blood sugar levels, and blood pressure, and is important in making protein, bone, and healthy DNA, as well as in decreasing the risk of bone fractures and aging from lack of movement. Levels of magnesium are also commonly deficient, so monitoring your blood levels of that mineral may be important.

What to be cautious about: More than 600 mg of calcium as a supplement can increase prostate cancer risk, and what is found for prostate cancer is usually found for breast cancer (and vice versa).[11] [12] And there is another special risk for women: Almost 70 percent of older females report taking calcium, but they may not know that more than 600 mg of calcium a day makes those who have had a stroke or who have white matter lesions (a marker for cerebrovascular disease) up to seven times more likely to develop dementia.[13]

How much to take: Do not take more than 600 mg as a supplement. Also, calcium from food affects the body differently than calcium from supplements and appears to be safe or even protective against vascular problems. So certainly if you've had a stroke, focus on these calcium-rich foods. You're aiming for 1,000 to 1,200 mg of calcium daily:

- One cup of nonfat cow's milk (276 mg) equals 23 percent of the recommended daily intake (RDI).
- One tablespoon sesame seeds has 9 percent of the RDI.
- One cup plain nonfat yogurt contains 30 percent of the RDI.
- Three ounces of canned salmon with bones equals 21 percent of the RDI.
- One cup cooked white beans has 13 percent of the RDI.
- One ounce of almonds contains 8 percent of the RDI.
- One cup cooked collard greens (226mg) equals 19 percent of the RDI.

DHA omega-3

Why you should take it: DHA, a component in fish oil, is a brain food. In randomized studies of people it has been found to help you stay healthier, and in a randomized controlled trial of people over the age of 60, it was shown to improve brain function, rendering benefits in speed of processing as if you were six years younger.[14] Taking omega-3 is also one of five practices that protect your eyes from the first phase of macular degeneration (the other four are ingesting the carotenoids lutein and zeaxanthin, avoiding cigarette smoke, and wearing sunglasses).[15]

What to be cautious about: We know of allergies to some fish-derived DHA. Be sure to get DHA rather than generic fish oils; many fish oil preparations do not contain the mostly active DHA. Also, recent data indicate a slight risk of atrial fibrillation from large doses of "fish oil." Nevertheless, the benefit exceeds the risk for most individuals over age 50. Talk to your doc about this.

How much to take: We suggest you take 900 mg daily or eat 12 to 16 ounces of wild salmon or 20 to 24 ounces of ocean trout a week: They are the only two fish in North America that consistently provide this key "fish oil." Or take algal (derived from algae) omega-3 DHA at a dose of at least 900 mg a day.

Low-dose aspirin

Why you should take it: If there is one longevity supplement that we recommend everyone over age 49 talk to their doc about, it's two 81-mg aspirin (*not* enteric/coated) daily. This dose protects against nine different cancers (including rectal, esophageal, liver, lung, and colon), as well as heart- and artery-related conditions such as stroke, impotence, and deep-vein thrombosis.[16] The benefits, if you include average values for cancer reduction, exceed the risks for the typical man over 35 and woman over 45.[17]

What to be cautious about: Gastrointestinal upset and bleeding can happen, so check with your doc before taking. On this regimen, make sure to have a half glass of warm water before and after each dose—as that decreases the GI side effects by over 70 percent—and take one in the morning and one in the evening, as the anti-inflammatory effect that helps protect you from cancer and arterial dysfunction lasts only 16 hours. Take aspirin consistently; if you forget it for two days, there's an increased risk of rebound: increased clotting in veins and blood vessels. And note that hormone replacements such as estrogen, progesterone, and testosterone all can increase clotting tendency—so talk with your doc about adding aspirin to this regimen. If you take aspirin, consider also taking 2,000 mg of bovine colostrum, as that decreases "leaky gut" and other GI symptoms from NSAIDs by about 80 percent.[18] There is also a liquid form of aspirin on the way to FDA approval, but we do not know if the reduction in side effects with the liquid form is greater than the benefit of bovine colostrum tablets.

How much to take: One baby aspirin (81 mg) each morning and night with half a glass of warm water before and after.

Omega-7

Why you should take it: Omega-7 fatty acids seem to decrease inflammation and insulin resistance, and thereby provide longevity benefits.[19]

What to be cautious about: We do not know of problems with this supplement unless it is not pure and contains the saturated version of palmitic acid (as do most preparations from sea buckthorn).

How much to take: We suggest 420 mg of purified omega-7 daily.

Probiotics

Why you should take it: Probiotics (the good-for-you bacteria in fermented food) help metabolize the youth- and energy-giving benefits in foods. Eating more than four ounces of red meat or six ounces of pork a week changes the bacterial makeup in your gut and produces chemicals that contribute to arterial aging, heart attack, and stroke.[20] [21] Avoiding these is sure to make you healthier for the long run. Decreased bacterial diversity in your microbiome is associated with aging.[22]

What to be cautious about: Getting this diversity from fermented foods is a great alternative as long as you eat them consistently. Over the next five to 10 years we expect to be able to recommend personalized probiotics for you.

How much to take: We advocate taking a daily supplement of either Lactobacillus GG or Bifidobacterium bifidum in spore form to increase the diversity of the bacteria in your gut (these forms survive your stomach acid). Or do as we do and alternate two or three choices (such as Culturelle, Digestive Advantage, or TruBiotics) at a dose of four billion live cultures or spore equivalents a day to try to increase diversity of your microbiome.

Coenzyme Q10

Why you should take it: This coenzyme works with other enzymes to foster your production of energy as you age.[23] It may also foster better brain function for your age reboot by reducing your risk of diabetes and hypertension. And according to two studies, it can decrease your risk of heart attacks, strokes, and all-cause mortality by substantial amounts. It seems to work by helping restore vigor to your mitochondria— the energy centers of each cell in your body. If you take LDL-lowering statins, atorvastatin and rosuvastatin, CoQ10 levels in your blood can decrease by 50 percent, so taking a supplement is a way to restore these levels.[24]

What to be cautious about: Statins do have substantial anti-inflammatory effects that benefit keeping your brain's arteries young, as well as those of your heart.[25] But 15 percent of people do have muscle soreness that is usually lessened by switching statins and adding CoQ10. We do not know of CoQ10 side effects that limit its use; patients with neurologic disease often take six times the recommendation for longevity without side effects greater than those seen in placebos.

How much to take: We recommend 200 mg daily (and if you are over 50, talk to your doc about a statin, especially if your LDL is above 70).

Avocado soybean unsaponifiables (ASU)

Why you should take it: A major way to improve longevity is to have a drug that keeps arthritis away. Since the 1990s, ASU has been prescribed in France for preventing arthritis. A large, three-year study from there, published in 2013 in the *British Medical Journal (BMJ)*, showed that 300 mg a day of ASU 300 significantly reduced progression of hip osteoarthritis compared with a placebo.[26] Saponification is the process of making soap from oil and lye; ASUs are one percent of the portion of the oil from avocados and soybeans that cannot be made into soap. ASU is also called A1S2 because it comes from a mixture of one part avocado oil and two parts soybean oil.

What to be cautious about: No serious side effects have been reported.[27]

How much to take: 300 mg daily.

NR (nicotinamide riboside) as the precursor to NAD (nicotinamide adenine dinucleotide)

Why you should take it: NR is believed to help with the function of mitochondria, which provide energy to your cells to help them function younger.[28][29] Most antiaging researchers at a 2019 conference indicated they were taking it (by a show of hands). It has reversed Alzheimer's in a mouse model, and helped restore muscle function in several models of muscle dysfunction with age. Many scientists think that lack of energy production by mitochondria is part of the major cause of some of the symptoms of aging, and that restoring NAD levels with a supplement such as Tru Niagen may help your mitochondria function as if they were years younger. Some say that it may at least keep your energy levels from declining further.

What to be cautious about: While we have good safety data in humans, we do not know if NR (Tru Niagen or an equivalent) has the same benefit in humans as it does in animals.

How much to take: No one is sure of the appropriate dose in humans, but 200 to 300 mg of NR seems to be the human equivalent dose that improved mitochondrial function in several animal species.

> While we think the data about the supplements above show that benefits are greater than risks for many people (do check with your caregiver), the supplements below need to be curated by your caregiver just for you, as each has benefits and risks that are not yet clear enough to make generalizations about risk-benefit calculations. Use our app or check GreatAgeReboot .com for more information on these.

Curcumin with bioperine

Why you should take it: Curcumin can help with cognitive function, which is especially important as you age. Curcumin with bioperine has been used to prevent the development of cognitive and functional decline and does so in animals and epidemiologic trials.[30] [31] The combo is undergoing small clinical human trials.

What to be cautious about: To date, there is no clear indication that these agents should be widely utilized in older adults pending further studies. The impact appears to be in its anti-inflammatory properties. Side effects of headaches have been reported.[32]

How much to take: 500 mg three times a day appears to be the human equivalent of the dosages used in animal studies done so far, and thus should have minimal side effects.

Metformin

Why you should take it: Metformin has been demonstrated in animal studies and in one epidemiologic human trial to improve longevity and decrease chronic disease burden.[33] [34]

What to be cautious about: There is concern that metformin eradicates the benefits of exercise, so while we recommend this to couch potatoes, it is not advocated for those who are physically active (though some are using it on days they do no exercise).[35] That contrasts substantially with our feelings about NAD (NR), which does not seem to have side effects or toxicity in humans. Low blood sugar can occur with metformin, and severe life-threatening acidosis has been reported in people who are dehydrated.[36] And some contamination that promotes cancer if very large doses are consumed has been reported in some generic versions.

How much to take: Large-scale clinical trials are under development at a dose of 500 mg of metformin twice a day, or 1,000 mg in the morning and 500 mg in the evening versus a placebo. Other supplements like creatine and n-acetylcysteine, and medications like rapamycin, potentially have greater benefit than risk in certain populations. Please consult your physician and our GreatAgeReboot.com app or website for more information on these and other supplements as data accumulate. We will try to keep the site as current as our scientific team can review and validate such data.

Self-Engineer Your Critical Eye

The internet is a wonderful thing—between the wealth of information at the tap of your fingers and the amazing videos of puppies curling up with ducks, what's not to love? But the downside is a lot of misinformation. While there's plenty of solid advice, good inspiration, and support groups in our digital world, you still have to tread carefully.

Consider this: A recent study looked at online symptom checkers.[37] While human doctors make misdiagnoses about 5 percent of the time (that's about 12 million U.S. adults annually, and more evidence that second opinions are worthwhile), misdiagnosis by digital tools happens 50 percent of the time.

And a 2019 study in the *BMJ* found that online tools made the correct diagnosis only 34 percent of the time. Better than zero, but not as good as actual doctors.

That underscores the importance of being a smart digital consumer. Use online information as one data point, and then use human input (i.e., your doctor and a second or third opinion) to help you determine problems and solutions.

Very often we use the anecdotal approach to medicine. *My friend had a friend who swore that eating three blueberries every morning reversed her diabetes.* Well, while blueberries are good, we're not so sure just three of them have that profound of an effect. This is a classic case of emotion in action. Most of us are more swayed by individual stories—and that can be a very good thing when it comes to inspiration—but perhaps we put too much stock in them as the only answer. Statistics can be complicated, but insightful.

That's why we want you to be critical consumers of medical and financial studies and reports. Knowing how they work will help you bust through the hype of headlines to figure out how a medical intervention should be considered. These are gold-standard terms that can be helpful to understand.

Observation: Done via epidemiological studies, observations give us insights into medical patterns by looking at populations and behaviors for an indication of some kind of variable at work. For example, let's say a study looked at a population of 50,000 people over a period of time, and each person had to report their eating patterns and health history. Once researchers controlled for all of the variables of eating patterns and health history, they could siphon out meaningful data. What if that study found that those who ate desserts more than five times a week had a 50 percent higher risk of having heart attacks? That's not a direct cause and effect. We don't know if, in fact, banana splits led to clogged arteries. But we do know there's a pattern that may offer some meaningful insight.

Intervention: After detecting a pattern, the question becomes: What helps? What action, device, medication, or other therapy stops or improves the biological mechanism that is causing the problem? This, as you can imagine, is a robust area of research. There are so many potential answers, especially depending on a research team's interest—be it diet, stress management intervention, or a pharmaceutical or some other solution. You have to look at what the study is telling you not just in terms of information, but also in terms of how rigorous that study was. Were variables controlled? Was it done on rats or humans? How many subjects were studied? Was the study supported by Big Pharma or by the National Institutes of Health? It's not always easy to decipher this information in a news report or a tweet, but it's worth a few minutes of sleuthing (many news stories link to the original article)—click any links to see if the data supports the news item.

Meta-analysis: This is a study that looks at the results of many studies, thus making it a comprehensive overview of the most important data out there. But the meta-analysis conclusion depends on the quality of studies used to make the meta-analysis. If you want to see if fish oil decreases heart attacks, the quality of the fish oil and the quantity each subject received and the control subjects' oil choices (did the control subjects get an oil that increases heart attacks?) are important to consider. Remember: garbage in, garbage out. If you look at

10 studies of 100 patients each, and they're poorly designed, the fact that you're analyzing 1,000 patients doesn't make the results any more reliable.

Double-blind, placebo-controlled: This type of study tries to ensure that the results and conclusions rule out a placebo effect and show some significance with the intervention. With the placebo effect, the subjects don't know whether they are receiving the trial medication or a placebo that tastes and looks and feels just like the medication. A problem here is if some or many of the subjects in the placebo group believe that aspirin is good and take it in addition to the placebo (they do this when they believe in the effect and "break" the study protocol, as 36 percent of participants did in one study). Sometimes the real story is buried deep within the data tables—which is why having a team help you interpret the news is so important.

Peer-reviewed: Because anything can be published on the internet, you want to make sure any studies you're relying on have gone through the rigor of peer review—that is, independent analysis by experts to validate the methods and procedures. But keep in mind that "peer-reviewed" is not "God-reviewed," as peers have their own biases.

Numbers: How many subjects were studied? Seven? That may not be very robust (unless perhaps all prior patients died but now six of the seven have survived after the new treatment). The higher the number, the more revealing the results, typically. Also realize that a 10 percent impact could, for example, be due to a 100 percent impact on 10 percent of the people or a 10 percent impact on everyone. They aren't the same result, but it is hard to determine which is the case.

SELF-ENGINEER YOUR APPEARANCE

If you feel a new sense of youthfulness, you may very well also thirst to *look* young. But the fact is, you almost inevitably gain some wrinkles as you get older. Scientists call this aging a "functional deterioration of the skin."

We asked our friend Arthur W. Perry, M.D., FACS, adjunct associate professor of surgery at Columbia University, to take us through some of the options for battling that deterioration. (See also DrPerrys.com for skin protection products and more information—he is a great doc, a skillful surgeon, and a science nerd who has done an amazing job in creating products that make you look younger.)

From face-lifts to tummy tucks, there are 1.8 million cosmetic surgery operations performed yearly in the United States. And "minimally invasive" (no scalpel needed) procedures—from laser hair removal to Botox to fillers—have boomed in popularity to about 16 million each year. And they do help make your skin's age look as young as your RealAge. We're doing our best to keep looking as young as we feel. Many office procedures are low risk and have short or no downtime, while surgery still exposes us to the risk of infections, bleeding, blood clots, and worse. Everyone has their own level of tolerable risk, so be sure to consider all possible complications and benefits and discuss possible procedures with your internist before venturing down this path.

Since these services are marketed directly to consumers without the filter of your family doctor, misrepresentation and even fraud are unfortunately not uncommon. So, let's try to make some sense of the information on the 411-million-plus plastic surgery web pages (just those in English) that vie for your hard-earned dollars.

Skin Care

Looking younger starts with not smoking and limiting unprotected sun exposure. But try as you might to protect your skin, it is programmed to thin at a rate of one percent per year after age 30. Despite the hype for products with CBD oil, charcoal, plant stem cells, and peptides, there's not much science in those supposed solutions. The list of ingredients that have been proved to help your skin look younger is really quite short, but does include vitamin A, vitamin C, fruit acids, and niacinamide (a vitamin).[38] The single most important skin care ingredient is micronized zinc sunscreen, which has been proved to slow skin aging and reduce skin cancers. We favor the mineral sunscreens—zinc oxide and titanium dioxide—because they sit on the surface of the skin and reflect ultraviolet light. We prefer zinc, as sweat can turn the titanium into a looks-dead-as-heck gray on your skin. The effectiveness of non-zinc or nontitanium sunscreens is considered unproved by the FDA; they may be toxic and interfere with hormones.[39] Sunscreen should be applied whenever the UV Index is over 3; you can check the index number on your smartphone every morning.

Your basic facial skin care regimen should include washing twice a day with a type of soap that has the same pH (acidity) as your skin (see "neutral pH" on the label). Use a washcloth for one of those cleanings to help exfoliate the dead cells that make your skin rough. Use a morning skin protector with an SPF of 15 and then feed your skin at night with the vampire vitamins—that's vitamins A and C, two great ingredients that help your skin but are destroyed by UV light (and actually can age it if applied during the day).

Beware of the tons of creams, potions, etc., that promise a restoration of youth in an afternoon or a week. It took decades for your skin to thin, and it's asking a lot from your body just to stall the process. Some "antiaging" products can make you look temporarily younger, but often this effect is caused by inflammation and subsequent edema (swelling) that temporarily hides wrinkles. Yes, they work for an evening, but they make your skin older over the long term. Another type of product with immediate effects but without inflammation contains silicones that flatten eyelid bags and wrinkles as they dry. This is more like makeup; when it's washed off, your wrinkles return. (We think Cinderella might have used this one.)

A few other important points: First, if the product makes claims that are too good to be true, those claims probably are bogus (let's face it: If it really did all that great stuff, the FDA would insist it be labeled as a prescription drug!). Second, if the jar you're considering costs more than a good dinner at your favorite restaurant, pass it up. (Even moisturizers, held in high esteem since Vaseline came out in 1870, have very little anti-aging science behind them. They can, though, help with dry skin.) Third, if you have atopic dermatitis or eczema, or if you have dry cracked skin caused by the weather or from washing too much, or from loss of hormones during menopause, moisturizers with ingredients like ceramides, emollients, and humectants (whew!) are reasonable treatments.

You can slow the aging process with carefully chosen skin care, but eventually, you'll sag and wrinkle. Fillers, peels, lasers, and botulinum toxins can help stave off wrinkles.

Noninvasive Techniques

Botulinum Toxin (You Can Call It Botox)

The only muscles in the body we don't recommend exercising are the ones in your face. That's because repeated flexing of the facial skin by the muscles underneath it eventually weakens that skin. You'll wake up one day and see a wrinkle, which really is a crack in the collagen layer.

Neurotoxins like Botox minimize wrinkles by halting the repeated muscle pull on the skin, which allows the wrinkles to actually heal and fill in. These drugs are the most potent toxins known to mankind; harnessed for good, they not only help you look better, but can actually make you happier (psychological studies have shown that people who can't frown feel better than those who can).

Botulinum injections are most useful for horizontal forehead wrinkles, "elevens" (the vertical wrinkles between the brows), and crow's-feet. They'll last about four months.[40]

Fillers

We prefer fillers to Botox to help "de-age" the lower face. Fillers have actually been around since the early 1980s, when collagen was borrowed from cows to help aging celebrities look younger. Today, the practice of injecting fillers has become an art form; skilled plastic surgeons and dermatologists use hyaluronic acid to fill facial and neck wrinkles and scars, build up cheekbones and chins, hide jowls, and flatten nasolabial folds and marionette lines, as well as to define, lift, and expand lips. (Yes, there is a cure for lipstick bleed!)

Filler is safest when used in the lower part of the face, since it can accidentally be injected into or absorbed into blood vessels. (This can be dangerous, since blood vessels in the upper face connect with important ones in the eyes and brain.) Additionally, fillers carry some rare risks, including blindness, stroke, and skin loss and the common risk of looking like a duck if the injections are performed by an unartistic doc (or maybe a veterinarian). About 50 people have gone blind from filler injections, so be careful when choosing your doc!

Newer versions of hyaluronic acid stick around for about a year and do more than just fill wrinkles. By stiffening skin, they stall the development of new wrinkles—and most interestingly, they fool your skin into thinking you're gaining weight so that it begins to generate more collagen.[41] This collagen generation is why there can be some permanence to wrinkle fillers; years later, chances are good that you'll look better.

High-Tech Options

Burning your face is hardly noninvasive, but different types of energy, like light, sound, and electricity all create controlled burns. Humans heal burns by shrinking and thickening skin: exactly what is needed to counter aging.[42] It may sound like it's from a *Saturday Night Live* skit, but literally hundreds of skin-burning machines have been created to help rejuvenate your face.

Lasers have been around for decades, but they still sound high tech. These devices can zap red capillaries, brown spots, and wrinkles. Old techniques that remove skin and create huge painful wounds have been replaced with "fractionated" lasering. CO_2 lasers do this most efficiently—check what laser type your practitioner uses—by drilling tiny holes in the skin (we'll wait for you to get up off the floor) that cause the shrinkage and thickening. The skin is left intact between the holes. You'll still have to hide for a few days after this treatment, but there's no painful wound. This "fractionated" technique, as opposed to the older ablative ("strip the skin") versions, can be done with just a topical anesthetic cream. With the laser and TCA (trichloroacetic acid) peels, you'll need to reserve about six days for hiding. You'll feel fine but look terrible until your skin flakes off, revealing lovely, even toned skin. Not for the faint of heart, deeper peels can turn back the clock by many years and the effects can last for decades.

Fractionated lasers require multiple treatments to smooth the skin, but they are particularly effective for those hard-to-treat cheek wrinkles.

Radio frequency (electric current) and microneedling have become popular, and there is some evidence that they help aging skin. But the science behind these techniques has been questioned by some. Radio frequency, along with lasers and high-energy ultrasound, are all "energy-generating machines." They create controlled burns that our bodies heal by—you guessed it—shrinking and thickening skin. If the treatments are done correctly, we look better. If done poorly, well, just watch the Oscars to see examples. Microneedling reminds us of those rototillers driving tiny needles into the skin to injure it and stimulate the wound-healing process to make it look younger. While there is some evidence that microneedling protects against some UV-caused skin aging, there is no standardization in the machines, and not a lot of scientific evidence documenting effectiveness and longevity of results. The best use of microneedling might turn out to be for stretch marks or for the types of scars that thin the skin.

High-energy focused ultrasound is a new way to rejuvenate the skin and is one of the few technologies that truly has zero downtime. Sound energy is focused and beamed for a fraction of a second under the skin, creating tiny wounds and stimulating the healing process. Ultherapy, as it is called, smooths crepey face, neck, and chest skin, and can subtly lift jowls and brows. After a single treatment, it takes three months to see the full effects, which then last about two years.[43] Ultherapy works best on thinner people and people physiologically (with RealAges) in their 50s and 60s.

Peels

Some chemicals can literally melt off your skin—and make it look better. The deeper the peel, the more profound the effect but the more downtime you'll have. Most useful for lighter skin types, peels can even out skin tone and remove splotchy pigmentation; deeper versions can smooth out wrinkles for decades. The choice of which peel to undergo depends largely on how much suffering you want to endure. Glycolic peels are for those who cannot take any time off to recover, or for people with darker skin, since deeper peels can cause splotchy results. These are performed by a dermatologist, a plastic surgeon, or a supervised nurse (we do not recommend that they be done by aestheticians, since the effects are variable enough that even superficial peels can burn some people). If your skin is discolored from all those weekends at the beach, the TCA (trichloroacetic acid) peel can erase most of those marks. This one must be performed by a physician, since it is easy to cause scarring. Deeper peels with phenol are still in use, but not nearly as popular as they once were, given their potential to create more toxicity.

Treatments for Wrinkled Chest Skin

Ultherapy—that high-energy focused ultrasound that is so useful on the face—also has been shown to smooth lines in the upper chest between the breasts, the décolletage. If those wrinkles are really deep, hyaluronic acid wrinkle filler can help here too. The laser is dangerous to use in this area because it can cause scarring, but intense pulsed light (IPL) can help by decreasing some of the splotchy pigmentation caused by too many trips to the beach. IPL requires many treatments that cost a few hundred dollars each, spaced a few weeks apart, to see its subtle, but real, effects.

"Thing" Removal

As we age, many "things" grow on the skin. Benign age spots (which are like freckles), raised seborrheic keratoses (which look like barnacles), moles (benign tumors of the pigment-producing cells, which can be raised or flat, brown, black, or even pink, with or without hair), skin tags, warts, premalignant actinic keratoses (these look like scrapes and overgrown or flaking skin), and even skin cancers sneak up on us as we age. A session at the plastic surgeon or dermatologist to shave, excise, freeze, or peel off these "things" can result in a remarkable improvement in appearance. Don't try and do this at home, since only a trained eye (or an AI system hooked to a large database, coupled with a trained eye) can decide which "thing" is really a cancer.

Surgical/Invasive Procedures

As aging progresses, skin care and noninvasive techniques eventually become less helpful. That's when we start considering real surgery. Eyelid-, brow-, and face-lifts (which involve varying levels of severity) all take years off your appearance. These usually require the removal of skin and some fancy tailoring, and are performed under local anesthesia with intravenous sedation. We strongly recommend an anesthesiologist to give you a little sedation and a lot of safety but try to avoid general anesthesia because of the increased risk of bleeding and blood clots in the legs with face-lift procedures.

Face-lifts

The noninvasive procedures such as fillers, botulinum, lasers, and peels can only go so far in preserving your youth. At some point, you may decide that a face-lift is the answer for you. But don't wait too long, because face-lifts performed in younger people (under 55, for instance) last longer and look better than if you wait until those crags are deeper than the Grand Canyon. There are as many face-lift techniques as there are plastic surgeons, but most lift the jowls in one layer and the skin in a second. New "short scar lifts" hide scars better because they eliminate the scarring above and behind the ear, and you won't lose hair. No matter how good your surgeon is, incisions within the hairline often cause damage to fragile hair follicles, so try to avoid those altogether. Men have a harder time with face-lifts, since most don't have long hair that can hide incisions.

Eyelid Lifts

Extra eyelid skin, from the fat that cushions your eyeballs eventually pushing outward, gives you a tired appearance. In this procedure, your doc numbs your eyelids and snips the extra skin. The surgical challenge is in not overdoing it and making you look strange. With a newer technique, your surgeon can lift your eyebrows above the bony rim without using forehead or scalp incisions. This "browpexy" gives a more natural look than the often overdone browlifts of the last generation. A medication (eye drops) has recently been approved to apply daily that seems to similarly (but temporarily) provide eyelid lifts.

Liposuction of the Neck and Jowls

As we grow older, our fat redistributes where we don't want it. Aging leaves cheekbones flat and the jawline indistinct. Worse, we get the dreaded "turkey gobbler" and neck bands. Liposuction, one of the biggest "bang for your buck" procedures, sucks fat out of the neck and jowls. Perennially one of the top two most popular procedures in cosmetic surgery, it can give the appearance of massive weight loss while tightening the neck skin; the fat-laden skin looks tighter because it drapes over a longer distance after suctioning. Despite the popularity of killing fat by freezing, heating, or melting it, the best proven method of defatting the neck is liposuction. This procedure can be completed in a little over an hour, with local anesthesia and light sedation. After some initial bruising, you'll be back in action in just a few days.

Rhinoplasty

An aging nose tip often sags and becomes bulbous. In rhinoplasty, a little incision is made between the nostrils and the skin is lifted up like the hood of a car, exposing cartilages and bones, which are then sculpted. Rhinoplasties in older people are more conservatively performed than the honker shrinkers that teenagers tend to have; bones are not usually broken, since they are so much more brittle as we age.

Hand Rejuvenation

Now that you have a 40-year-old face, what about those 70- to 100-year-old hands? In the last decade plastic surgeons have figured out how to rejuvenate aging hands. Thin crepey skin exposes tendons and blood vessels. Filler, usually white calcium hydroxylapatite (Radiesse), hides those structures while the CO_2 laser helps crinkled, splotchy skin. Lasering the hands takes only a few minutes, and usually the forearms are included so that no brown/white line is seen. Some surgeons excise visible veins on the back of the hands, but we feel this is not a good idea, since sooner or later, you'll need those veins for a medical procedure.

Body Rejuvenation

Breast Surgeries

Aging breasts sag and shrink after pregnancy. Silicone implants are the most common form of cosmetic surgery— but women should think carefully about getting these after age 40, since they can interfere with mammogram interpretation and accuracy. If you have implants, you'll need an MRI at least every year to stay safe. Worse, a rare risk of implants is a mouth bender called breast implant–associated anaplastic large cell lymphoma (BIA-ALCL); one in 30,000 women with textured implants develop this cancer, which has prompted some countries to consider banning this type of implant.[44] As bad as it sounds, the problem is usually removed and cured with surgery (the cancer and implant are both removed). Much study is needed to better understand this condition.

Another common cosmetic breast procedure is mastopexy, also known as a breast lift; the nipples are raised and extra skin removed to give breasts their youthful shape. There's also reduction mammoplasty, which makes large breasts (which can cause back and neck pain, along with yeast rashes in warm weather) smaller, using the same type of incisions as those used in lifts. Cosmetic breast surgery is usually an outpatient procedure done under general anesthesia. You'll be back to work and play in just a few days.

Tummy Tucks

Your babies and too many chocolate glazed doughnuts along the way did a number on your belly; as a result, you've got stretch marks, your posture worsens, and your back aches. That's all because the belly muscles—the ones that create a six-pack—drift to the sides during pregnancy (and can do the same in men who have "beer bellies"). Tummy tucks fix those muscles and remove extra skin and fat. Best of all, this is a "four for one" procedure because not only will you look better after surgery, you'll feel better, stand up straighter, and have stronger abdominal muscles. This surgery is done under general anesthesia and generally doesn't require a hospital stay. You'll have a few annoying drains sticking through the incision for a few days, and it will hurt when you get out of bed, but your shape will dramatically change. That said, you've got to be healthy to have a tummy tuck; there's a real risk of bleeding and even life-threatening blood clots. And don't even think about having this operation if you're a smoker since the rate of complication, including disastrous loss of skin, is much higher for tobacco users.[45]

Liposuction

Mr. Dyson wishes he had thought of this procedure, which vacuums out fat from the belly, hips, or thighs and even other more unusual locations like the back under the bra line, your cankles, and chubbs (that's the knees for those of you who don't watch reality TV). Once the fat is removed through tiny incisions, the skin usually shrinks. If you already have stretch marks or hanging skin, you won't attain the needed shrinkage (which just won't happen if it is already stretched that far); that means liposuction is not the correct procedure for you. Keep in mind that this is not a method of weight loss; it's a way to contour discrete fat deposits you'd rather not have. As long as you don't overdo it, it's a very safe procedure. The rule of thumb is that if you need more than 10 pounds suctioned, you should lose weight before considering liposuction.

Brazilian Butt Lift

Neither Brazilian nor an actual butt lift, this poorly named procedure expands the buttocks by taking fat from your belly and injecting it into your derriere, creating the effect of a rounded, aesthetically appealing rear end. Nevertheless, the results are often deadly; in fact, 3 percent of board-certified plastic surgeons who conducted this procedure have had a patient die on them, often due to fat getting into the bloodstream and clogging the lungs.[46] We wish American plastic surgeons would ban this crazy procedure—other countries have already done so. Instead, we recommend lunges, squats, and other buttock exercises to improve the appearance of your glutes.

Cellulite Reduction Treatment

Nope, there's just no proven drug, food supplement, or cream that can alleviate cellulite. Every few years, a machine is introduced that promises to get rid of it—but once swelling goes away, it often returns. If the dimples are deep enough, they can be filled with fat taken from another part of the body. But at this time, we can't in good faith recommend any particular treatment to reduce cellulite.

CHAPTER 15

SELF-ENGINEERING YOUR GREAT AGE REBOOT

How to jump-start your longevity plan

We hope that by now you have learned the absolute importance of self-engineering your DNA switches—that is, directing your future by turning your genes on or off through good lifestyle choices.

How are you going to prepare for the intersection between what the medical community can do for you and what you can do for yourself?

We suggest a five-step process of preparation. But you can and should customize that process. There may be some things that you have a good handle on already (good for you if you're in excellent health and/or have been a prudent saver!). But that doesn't mean you stop. You should always be thinking about how your life and your circumstances may change.

Things change as you age. Things change as life throws curveballs. Things change because society changes.

Therefore, these suggestions aren't meant to be a static plan that will guarantee good health and high wealth. They are intended to help you take stock of where you are and want to be. Outlining your current status, along with your goals, your dreams, and your vision, allows you to make the best use of the action steps outlined in this book.

The process of rebooting is a three-legged stool:

Advancing medical knowledge and treatments that keep us healthier longer. This is in the hands of researchers, doctors, hospitals, and artificial intelligence. They will proceed without our help to take advantage of new knowledge.

Ensuring economic security. You'll need to work and save the fruits of your labor to enjoy your longer, prosperous, and happier life.

Making a life. If we are healthy, able to work, and can handle our finances well, we will make a living. But we also need to make a life! Each of us will have many decisions to make involving the heart, the mind, and the soul.

These five actions will help you find *your* way, no matter what your age.

WHAT'S COMING: Data Will Dictate Decisions
WHAT TO DO: Collect Yours

No matter what changes are first, what changes are widespread, and what changes you will take advantage of, one thing is certain: Data will inform what will work best for you. These data will come from things that you can't (yet!) do on your own but that you can get with help from your team (genetic testing, blood tests, etc.), which underscores an important tenet:

- To use your data to make good decisions, you must collect it. Your data measures will give you an indication of where your strengths lie, as well as which areas need improvement.

One caution: While these numbers can be emotionally charged (if, for example, you get depressed over the number on the scale or in your retirement account), you have to let your logic override your emotions and let the data point to the places where work needs to be done. The next step? Getting the data to where you want it.

Activity: Create a file (either a spreadsheet or a journal) that includes your starting point numbers (see the template below). Some numbers you will have handy; some you may need to access (perhaps with a visit to your doctor or to your online medical chart). Take an afternoon to record them, and follow up with a yearly inventory, so you can track changes over time.

HEALTH

Age: _____

Weight: _____

Blood pressure (aim <125/<85): _____

Waist circumference (aim less than half your height in inches): _____

Blood sugar (aim <98 mg/dL): _____

LDL cholesterol (aim <70 mg/dL): _____

HEALTH

Advanced credit:

APO B (aim <80 mg/dL): _____

Lipoprotein A (aim <30mg/dL): _____

hsCRP (aim <1.0): _____

Il-6 (aim <1.8pg/mL): _____

TMAO (aim <2 uM/L): _____

MPO (aim <470 pmol/L): _____

Regular credit:

Smoke or vape (aim never): _____

Do you practice stress management (aim=YES): _____

Immunizations up-to-date: _____

Last eye exam: _____

Last hearing exam: _____

Last olefactory (smelling) exam: _____

Last bone mineral density test: _____

Last PAP or prostate exam: _____

Last colonoscopy: _____

Extra credit:

Max heart rate during max exercise: _____

Heart rate decrease in 2 mins after stop of max exercise of 20 mins of cardio: _____

Are you doing the skin preservations recommended in Chapter 14?: ___

Are you doing the brain games recommended in Chapter 13?: _____

Are you taking the supplements recommended in Chapter 14?: _____

WEALTH

Yearly income: _____

Retirement account: _____

Value of other assets: _____

Debt (credit card and other): _____

Are you putting away 10 percent of your gross income in a retirement account?: _____

How diversified is your savings portfolio?: _____

WHAT'S COMING: Your Inner Circle Will Become Even More Vital
WHAT TO DO: Build Your Team

Creating a buddy system may very well be one of the most vital practices you can put in place right now. That's because social support is one of the most influential factors on health (this applies not just to obvious scenarios like depression, but also for age-related illnesses like dementia). And if the pandemic of 2020 taught us nothing else, it was that we must make efforts to maintain connections, even during times when we physically can't be present.

This buddy system isn't just to identify a pickleball partner. It's to make sure that you have social, medical, financial, and logistical teams in place to help you manage your reboot and everything that comes with it. As medicine advances, you will need more people to help triangulate information and make decisions because there will be so many more choices and options, as each will be keeping up with more info in a smaller and smaller area. That goes for making decisions about cutting-edge treatments as well as for the interpersonal challenges that come when making hard choices.

One guideline we like: When you're younger, you want docs and financial experts who are older and have more experience. But when you're older, you want those docs to be younger—so they're more likely to be up on the latest advances and techniques and will be able to stay with you for the next 25 or 30 years.

Team building isn't just something you check off the list, but something you're constantly evaluating.

Activity: Think about the four pillars of your team. Write down existing members. If you're lacking in certain areas, think about what you will do to help build them. Also realize that these teams will morph as you age—and being fluid about maintaining social connections is one of the greatest skills you can have.

Medical (primary docs, specialists)	Financial (accountant, investment advisers)	Familial (biological and nonbiological)	Social (wider circles and connections)

WHAT'S COMING: Financial Security Will Fortify You in a Changing World
WHAT TO DO: Save, Save, Save

It's the number one thing you can do: Save, save, and save some more. It's one thing to say it; it's another to do it. And we certainly see the importance of that when the economy experiences a major downturn, as with the recession in 2008 and the massive economic downturn in the 2020 pandemic. Future medical advances may mean that you'll be healthier and can work longer, but having financial security will help protect you against inevitable dips in the economy.

Saving today is synonymous with spending tomorrow and there will be a lot of tomorrows. Save every week, even when you are not making much. Save even more as you make more. Plan to save 10 percent of your income all your life, and ask yourself if you can afford to save even more. If so, you will be more secure later in life, and free of financial stress. Your savings rate should rise faster than your income. This means controlling your urge to splurge when you get a big bonus (save it to tide you over in the year when you get no bonus!). Every time your income increases, put a larger incremental share—perhaps 20 percent of that increase—into savings. After all, you were living comfortably before the raise.

Remember, a healthy body doesn't mean squat if you have serious financial stress. And the reverse is true, too: Excellent money is no fun if your health is poor. Some important saving advice to get you started:

- While headlines tout eye-watering returns by hedge fund and private equity legends, most of us have neither the skill nor the infrastructure to attempt such strategies. Research shows that for almost all of us, the best route is to be well diversified in no-load, low-fee index funds. Every dollar saved in fees today is eight dollars in 42 years at a 5 percent annual return.

- Always be "in the market"—and do not pretend you know when to get in and out, since you do not know. Moving in and out creates needless fees, taxes, and losses. And as long as the money supply keeps increasing, some of that increased money will fuel the markets and economy.

- Debt is fun—until you have to pay it back at the worst possible time. So, as an alternative, live within your means. Do not count on a bonus or raise to cover your spending. Assume they will not happen—but if they do occur, have a celebratory meal and save most of the rest. People fall into the trap of borrowing from one lender or credit card to pay another. If you are doing that, stop now before it's too late. Cut your spending. We enjoy, but do not need, much of what we buy. Prioritize spending patterns and say no to yourself and your family. It will reduce financial stress and help you support a comfortable life in retirement.

Activity: Write down your current saving strategy. Now analyze your expenses and think about things you can cut out of your life on a monthly basis to direct more money to retirement and other savings accounts. Then, make a commitment to directly feed more money (via your paycheck) to those retirement accounts. This isn't always an easy choice—but it's easily one of the most important choices you can make.

Expense	Monthly Money Saved	Yearly Contribution (12x)
1.		
2.		
3.		

WHAT'S COMING: Advances Will Cure and Heal, but You Can Avoid Treatment With Nature's Medicine
WHAT TO DO: Reboot Your Approach to Food

We have medicine that can help with diabetes and cholesterol, and we may someday have meds that can repair stem cells or replace brain cells. But many docs will tell you that the way to avoid needing those meds in the first place is to take advantage of what the world has already provided for you.

Food is nature's fuel and medicine, and many of us are poisoning ourselves with too many calories—and too many of the wrong kinds of calories. We've covered the best foods to eat throughout this book: fish, vegetables, and healthy fats.

Of course, it isn't always easy to change your usual diet, especially if you've ignored healthy eating in the past. But you can start. One of the best ways to achieve this is through the idea of substitution—not necessarily taking something away, but finding a replacement for it. So instead of soda, can you switch to seltzer water with fruit in it? Instead of dessert every night, could you limit it to two nights a week and fill the other five nights with a bowl of berries?

Activity: Write down three of the foods or eating habits that may be contributing to bad health. Write down foods or activities that you could substitute to help replace the unhealthy habit with a healthy one.

Habit/Food	Substitute
1.	
2.	
3.	

WHAT'S COMING: The Changes Will Be Coming Fast
WHAT TO DO: Embrace Resilience

Adapting a new outlook on longevity is about playing the long game. There's no easy path to a long and happy life, and while that notion can be difficult to embrace in our quick-fix, fast-typing, scroll-through-social-media culture, it's the truth. When it comes to medical advances, there's a good chance that you will have many choices, you will be confused, you will not know what to trust, and you may not be able to tell the difference between snake oil and real elixirs. So part of managing the Great Age Reboot is having the right mindset to handle change.

You have to have some patience, and you have to give yourself some latitude when it comes to struggles, stresses, and enduring what is ahead. Life is more of a marathon than a sprint, and that's why endurance, resilience, and heart are more important than speed. Over the years, these are some of the guiding philosophies we have tried to live by:

- Life is not easy. It becomes easier when you have close and loving friends, companions, a life partner, and, above all, a community to help you through both good times and bad times.

- Plan your life, but remember most things that happen to you are things you did not plan. Example: How did you meet your spouse, significant other, and friends, select your college, your job, or the city in which you live?

- You do not choose the things that happen to you, but you always get to choose how to deal with them. So, if you have high blood pressure, get it under control with life-style or medication now.

- Do not get hung up on the past. Your life is made up of the present and future, and your past helps you navigate.

- There is no limit to what you can accomplish if you don't care who gets the credit—which means you always must work with others and share the wins and the losses.

- Love others as you wish to be loved. All of us are better off when we learn from others. We live in a knowledge-centered world; keep learning!

- As you go through life, make this your goal: Keep your eye upon the doughnut and not upon the hole. (And don't eat the doughnut!)

Activity: Write down the most important "life mantras" you have. These will be your guiding principles and values; they'll help you make big and small decisions every day and will go a long way in helping you improve your overall happiness.

ACTIVITY

_____

_____

_____

_____

_____

_____

CRUCIAL AGE-RELATED DECISIONS THAT MAKE YOU 20-PLUS YEARS YOUNGER

If You're in Your 20s or Early 30s
About Your Health

Genetics: It's important to know your genetic risk factors (you can use ancestry programs and many family history programs and apps as a template to help you understand the right questions to ask). Understand your risk factors and talk to your primary doc. And realize that you can change these risks through your behaviors.

Toxins: Avoid them. Abandon all tobacco (cigarettes, pipes, cigars). The pleasure now just isn't worth the future heart and other pains. If you use marijuana, eat it rather than smoke it (and protect it and all medications or other substances from children and unexpected guests who just might open your medicine cabinet when using your bathroom). Pick a living and working space as far from active motorways as possible. And wash your hands before you eat anything and after using public facilities. Please.

Chef skills: Learn to properly cut vegetables, which may be the single simplest thing you can do to help your health because it encourages you to integrate more disease-fighting veggies into your life. What Dr. Mike found after working with thousands of people is that if you invest in a high-quality knife and learn how to use it quickly and efficiently, your time savings in meal preparation are enormous—and that exponentially increases your desire and willingness to make delicious meals with foods you love that love your body back.

About Your Money

Education: Each year of additional education has historically generated about a 7 percent annual return on average. But it is an investment that requires more than just showing up. Research shows that not all schools and fields of study have the same return. Education, like playing guitar, requires hard work. It is nice to pursue what you like, but if it does not provide a path to take care of yourself, it is a hobby. Some fields of study are interesting and fun but provide no obvious career path. You harm your financial life if you borrow $100,000 to work in a (perhaps interesting and noble) field where you will realistically earn $20,000 a year, as more than half of your gross income will need to go to repay your debt over 10 years.

Backup plans: Many people decide to take care of their families rather than work outside the home for pay. This may be done for a few months, or it may be a 20- to 25- year commitment. In a world full of divorces, you must consider from your first day out of the work-for-pay world how you will support yourself if separation occurs. That may include working in the family/childcare field using the skills you have developed. But it may also mean acquiring additional skills that would be marketable in work scenarios outside the home. Such contingency planning will better prepare you for the shocks of life.

If You're 35 to 60
About Your Health

Habits: In this whole quest to figure out how to make meaningful changes to your health and wealth, you can (yes, can) break bad habits and form good ones. It really is all about creating a life rhythm—an underlying beat to your life that is the foundation on which you form those good habits, make decisions, and build an automatic lifestyle of good health and strong wealth.

About Your Money

Investments: Use tax-deferred investment accounts as much as possible to improve your rate of return. Money invested in a tax-deferred account grows faster as the income earned is not taxed until the money is withdrawn years from now. And not having to pay the Internal Revenue Service is a good thing, as better you should have the money working for you than it being blown by D.C. In addition, about half of all employers will match your retirement saving in tax-deferred plans. Also, the adage "Do not put all of your eggs in one basket" is true of investing, even if it is a really good basket. All too often, people fall in love with a popular company (often the company for which they work) and put most of their money in its stock. But great companies eventually stumble, many quickly and dramatically. Diversified index funds with no load and low fees guarantee slightly above mediocre long-term returns. And that is pretty good over time. Some broad stocks, index funds, some real estate indexes, some bond indexes, perhaps your home, and perhaps a bit of gold give you a diversified portfolio. Research shows that no-load, low-fee index funds (and exchange-traded funds, or ETFs) provide the best long-term returns for investors.

Education: Be realistic about your children and their abilities. Are they college material or college drop-out material? If they go to college, will you be buying them an education or a holiday and drinking campaign? Are your children taking a well-rounded course load that will prepare them for the real world? If not, stop supporting their college efforts and save for your retirement.

If You're 60 to 80-Plus
About Your Health

Diet: Go to plant-based eating (except for salmon) and eat only when the sun is up. The alternation between ketosis from not eating when the sun isn't up and refeeding with great food is postulated (with quite a bit of animal and human evidence) to help throw several genetic switches—first into survival mode, where you harvest your old cells, and then into growth mode, where you repopulate with young cells. This style of eating can make you over 13 years younger by itself. The five food felons to avoid: trans fats, saturated fats (they come with proteins that change your microbiome), simple sugars, added syrups, and carbs stripped of nutrients (they raise your blood sugar too fast, though someday soon you'll be able to monitor your blood sugar moment to moment and keep it safely below 99 mg/dL).

Games: Reasoning or memory games only help your ability to reason or remember. The games that prevented dementia in three randomized controlled studies of people over age 70 were speed-of-processing games. Just 18 hours of practice over 10 years decreased the incidence and prevalence of dementia by over 25 percent, and increased neurotransmitter production and release in key brain areas.

About Your Money

Work: If you are enjoying work, why quit? And if you want to work a bit less, is there a way to scale back but continue to work for pay? The income reduces financial stress and you can keep saving for your longer expected life. It also keeps you connected to the world of today in terms of activities and technology. Plus, it provides a social framework. Assess what your income would be if you retire now and live on your resources without running down your savings. What spending pattern is supportable? Be realistic; you're old enough to no longer believe in fairy godmothers. If you cannot afford your desired spending pattern, either keep working and saving or reassess your desired spending to fit reality. Or better yet, do both!

Volunteering: You can do great social good with your time, knowledge, and money. Think of the transformed Scrooge in Dickens's *A Christmas Carol.* It is life transforming to be part of something good and bigger than us. It will also give you connectivity with people of other ages and will set the stage to replenish "your team" as members disappear.

Estate: Have a will that clearly delineates the disposition of your resources. Address and regularly revisit the hard questions. How much goes to charity versus loved ones? Which charities? Do loved ones share equally? How much will go to your children (biological or nonbiological), grandchildren, and great-grandchildren? How much to those loved ones who are well off, and to those with drug problems? We recommend that you revisit your wishes every two years with a lawyer for an hour or so, revising your will as your life and priorities evolve.

AFTERWORD

A Note About COVID-19

When COVID-19 hit the world in early 2020, we had just completed the first draft of this book. That meant we had spent more than a year researching, talking, strategizing, and thinking about health, immunity, and medical advances, which longevity gains were likely to occur, and what this phrase meant: "Longevity will be the greatest disruptor."

The pandemic forced us to question the two worlds we had been addressing—medical and financial. What would happen to our health and well-being? What would happen to our financial security?

The pandemic has taken a massive toll on our society in lives lost, money lost, and the way we view our own mortality. It has also spotlighted the way science and medicine can adapt, adjust, and search for solutions to problems we may not have expected to encounter but are indeed our new reality.

The world changed, yes, but something that didn't change was the main theme of this book—that YOU still own a large amount of control over your health destiny. Consider this statistic: In over 70 percent of all COVID-19 deaths, other conditions like diabetes, obesity, high blood pressure, cancer, or other immune deficiency or cardiovascular disease were present or the person was over 70 calendar years of age.[1] And those factors (except your calendar age) are things that largely can be controlled with lifestyle changes. That doesn't make the losses less significant. But it does reveal something vital: You have some control over even things that feel uncontrollable.

As you've seen, you can take advantage of all of the medical advances coming our way by being as healthy as possible. But COVID-19 also forced us to think about the flip side: You can protect yourself against threats we may not see coming—even before modern medicine can catch up—by fortifying your body the best that you can.

We know that COVID-19 changed your life in some way—whether it was with the loss of a loved one or the loss of a job or having to adjust the way you work and interact with people.

Whatever lessons and experience you took from the pandemic, our hope is that another key lesson is one you can apply to the Great Age Reboot: We are living in a dynamic world—a world in which you will have new opportunities and will need to make new decisions about your medical future. Your ability to adjust—and take care of yourself in the process—will dictate how long, well, healthy, and young you live.

14 SERIOUSLY SEMI-SERIOUS PREDICTIONS FOR 2050 AND BEFORE

1.	You will be able to replace body parts (except your brain) using your own stem cells and 3D printing.
2.	Many, maybe most, cancers will be able to be cured (not survived, but cured).
3.	We'll regularly see people live to 150.
4.	The average retirement age will be 75 or older.
5.	Giannis Antetokounmpo will still be playing in the NBA, along with his son. And maybe a grandson will be raring to go, too.
6.	When you look in a mirror, it will show you your vital signs and identify any suspicious skin marks, then report the data to your master medical portal, which will be immediately reviewed by your health and wellness team.
7.	As part of an annual physical, not only will you have your blood tested, but you will also have an annual fat-replacement procedure—brown fat for white fat—if needed.
8.	The Supreme Court will consider whether the laws passed by Congress regarding medical advances that bring children into the world through scientific and mechanical means are constitutional.
9.	Headlines will be filled with claims that the wealthy and healthy boomers are tired of supporting their millennial children, who are now in their 70s and are still asking their parents to pay for their communication (phone) bills.
10.	Housing will be much more communal: large buildings featuring private bedrooms and bathrooms, with common living spaces.
11.	Eyeballs will have night-vision and telephoto settings.
12.	We'll be excited (not fearful) about old age—because we will be much healthier every step of the way.
13.	Through cell and gene manipulation, we'll be able to create newborns to our exact specifications.
14.	Antiaging tacos!

ACKNOWLEDGMENTS

The authors would like to thank the incredible team at National Geographic for all of their work, commitment, and passion for turning our concepts into an accurate and spectacularly provocative reality. Hilary Black and Lauren Purcell persisted and brilliantly guided the writing and organization to make this book a much better reflection of what we hoped to share with readers. Without their dedication, you wouldn't be holding what we truly believe will be your go-to resource for understanding longevity and its implications for you and your family. Project manager Moriah Petty kept us on time—a timeline that was hugely impacted by the pandemic. In addition, our deepest appreciation goes to Lisa Thomas, Melissa Farris, Nicole Miller Roberts, Judith Klein, Kim Lewis, Daneen Goodwin, Ann Day, and Marisa Larson.

From Michael F. Roizen

The books I write are always secondary to my goal of helping people live longer, healthier lives—and that has only happened with the help of literary agent, super editor, and thought leader Candice Fuhrman. Thank you for so much, Candice! I also so appreciate the entire Nat Geo team, listed above, who worked on this project. A special thank you goes to Hilary Black, who tolerated my crazy concern about the cover as well as each paragraph. She was not only an exceptionally superb editor, but also oversaw the whole project and challenged us to make it the best it could be. Her thoughtful leadership made this book possible. Many thanks also go to Nat Geo's former editorial director Susan Goldberg for her deep support of this book—and its message.

Of course, this entire endeavor would not have been possible without my family members—especially the support, encouragement, and incisive comments of Dr. Nancy, my wonderful saint of a wife. Jen, the family chemist, and Jeff, the family pediatric endocrinologist, have contributed much encouragement as well. My wife's late 101+-year-old mother, Marion, demonstrated that aging can be a very vibrant time; her influence is squeezed into this book, as is that of my sister Marsha and brother-in-law Richard Lowry as critical readers. These direct family were joined at times by the "extended family" of the Katzes, Unobskeys, and Campodonicos. I would also like to thank Mehmet and Lisa Oz and their family, including Daphne; John Mauldin; Zack Wasserman; and others for encouraging and critiquing the concepts here.

This book would not have been possible without the long talks that bracketed weekly Ping-Pong games with co-author Albert Ratner (as well as frequent input from his wife and partner, Audrey). I hope the final product does justice to his humor and brilliance. I also was greatly motivated by co-author Peter Linneman's clear and concise economic analyses.

All of us were inspired by members of the Great Age Reboot company advisory board: Drs. Pat Cox, Nicola Finley, Louis Malinow, Larry May, Harry Oken, Julien Bailes, Nick Genes, Robert Colton, and Usha Satish. They all built on the foundation created by the co-workers, clinicians, scientists, and experts at the Cleveland Clinic, as well as co-workers in the Wellness Institute, who taught me that "Longevity Is the

Next Disruptor"™. Mladen Golubic, M.D., Ph.D., has always encouraged scientific rigor and deserves much of my applause. Thanks, too, to outside experts in longevity, but especially Drs. Shai Efrati, Peter Attia, Peter Diamandis, and David Sinclair. And we could not have done it without the team that has helped to create the Great Age Reboot Company, app, website, podcasts, and more: Rafhael Cedeno, Corey Bridges, John Day, Randall Myeroff, Craig Cogut, and board chair David Abramson.

Also important, I am fortunate to work with many caregivers who have broken traditional molds and are making the Cleveland Clinic the best place to work and the best place to receive care—especially if you desire wellness as both a culture and a long-term outcome. Our CEO took the position that our organization cannot continue to focus just on treating illness and caregiving to be a great institution. CEO Toby Cosgrove has observed, and new CEO Dr. Tom Mihaljevic has even more adamantly stated, that while the clinic is already known as one of the best for treating illness, wellness is also part and parcel of what we do for every employee and every person we touch.

Especially important was Wellness Operations director Percy Bhathena, chief coach Amy Gannon, and chief nutritionist Kristin Kirkpatrick. I want to thank all of them for their scientific contributions and constructive criticisms, and for allowing me the time and encouragement to complete this work. And I am fortunate to have worked over the last few years with the talented and creative group that includes Dr. Martin Harris, Dr. Bridget Duffy, Dr. Mike O'Donnell, Dennis Kenny, Dr. Rich Lang, Dr. Raul Seballos, Dr. Steven Feinleib,

Dr. Barbara Messinger-Rapport, Dr. Roxanne Sukol, and Dr. Rich Cartabuke. I would also like to thank Mike Kessel, Mira Ilic, Karen Tabor, Karen Jones, Dr. Jim Young, and the Canyon Ranch experts, including Dr. Rich Carmona, who run the gamut from inner-city schoolteachers (thank you, Rosalind Strickland) to those who inspire (thank you, Reverend Otis Moss).

The list of those who contributed to this book scientifically is also long. Special thanks go to Keith Roach and the late Anita Shreve, as well as the many gerontologists and internists who read sections of the book for accuracy. I would also like to recognize others on the RealAge team who validated and verified the content and contributed their expertise to the book.

My administrative associate Jackie Frey made this work possible, and the references were made more accurate by Grace Titgemeier. It's no accident that *U.S. News & World Report* has ranked the Cleveland Clinic number one in cardiac care 27 years in a row. My prior associate, Anne-Marie Prince, deserves special thanks, as does Diane Reverand—she started this process by telling me not to worry about offending medical colleagues. As long as the science was solid, she said, they would understand that we were trying to motivate *you* to understand that you can control your genes.

And, of course, Ted Spiker made writing much more accurate and enjoyable. I cannot say enough about how fantastic Ted is (yes, I ended that sentence with a verb, I know, I know).

I hope and believe this book will help readers live younger and longer. The notion that many more people could avoid confronting illness within our medical system for longer would be a physician's greatest reward.

From Peter Linneman

This book has been an enlightening learning experience. I would like to thank Dr. Lucille G. Ford for instilling in me the joy of constantly learning and growing, a process that I began 52 years ago. She is also the embodiment of productively aging as she approaches her 101st birthday. I also would like to thank my long-time friend and co-author Albert Ratner, who encouraged a somewhat skeptical me to join him and Michael on this adventure. And I thank my co-author Michael for constantly answering my endless questions.

From Albert Ratner

To Audrey, my wife, and to the Cleveland Clinic, both of whom have inspired my desire to ensure healthy longevity for others. Also thanks to Michael, Peter, and Ted for allowing me to add my experience to their skills and brilliance.

SOURCES

INTRODUCTION

1. Singapore University of Technology and Design, "Print Me an Organ: Why Are We Not There Yet?" *ScienceDaily* (2019). www.sciencedaily.com/releases/2019/12/191211082709.htm.

2. Adam Hoffman, "Tiny Robots Can Clear Clogged Arteries," *Smithsonian Magazine* (2015), https://www.smithsonianmag.com/innovation/tiny-robots-can-clear-clogged-arteries -180955774/.

3. Mingtao Zhang, Emily A. Eshraghian, Omar Al Jammal et al., "CRISPR Technology: The Engine That Drives Cancer Therapy," *Biomedicine & Pharmacotherapy* 133 (2021), doi: 10.1016/j.biopha.2020.111007.

4. Sarah K. Madden, Aline Dantas de Araujo, Mara Gerhardt et al., "Taking the Myc Out of Cancer: Toward Therapeutic Strategies to Directly Inhibit c-Myc," *Molecular Cancer* 20, article no. 3 (2021), doi:10.1186/s12943-020-01291-6.

5. David A. Sinclair and Matthew D. LaPlante, *Lifespan: Why We Age—and Why We Don't Have To* (New York: Thorsons, 2019).

6. Michael F. Roizen, *RealAge: Are You as Young as You Can Be?* (New York: Harper Collins, 1999).

7. Yasuyosh Ouchi, Hiromi Rakugi, Hidenori Arai et al., on behalf of the Joint Committee of Japan Gerontolgical Society and Japan Geriatrics Society on the Definition and Classification of the Elderly, "Redefining the Elderly as Aged 75 Years and Older: Proposal From the Joint Committee of Japan Gerontological Society and the Japan Geriatrics Society." *Geriatrics Gerontology International* 17, no. 7 (2017), doi:10.1111/ggi.13118.

8. William C. Hittinger, "Metal-Oxide-Semiconductor Technology," *Scientific American* 229, no. 2 (1973): 48–59, doi:10.1038/scientificamerican0873-48.

9. Michael F. Roizen and Mehmet C. Oz. *YOU: Losing Weight: The Owner's Manual to Simple and Healthy Weight Loss* (New York: Free Press, 2011).

10. Dana Goldman. "The Economic Promise of Delayed Aging," *Cold Spring Harbor Perspectives in Medicine* 6, no. 2 (2016): a025072, doi:10.1101/cshperspect.a025072.

11. CDC/NCHS, "Life Expectancy at Birth, at 65 Years of Age, and at 75 Years of Age, by Race and Sex: United States," *Vital Statistics Rates in the United States* (2010), https://www.cdc.gov/nchs/data/hus/2010/022.pdf.

PART 1
INTRODUCTION

1. "Life Expectancy in Industrial and Developing Countries in 2020." *Statista Research Department*, (Nov. 27, 2020). https://www.statista.com/statistics/274507/life-expectancy-in -industrial-and-developing-countries/.

2. Theresa Andrasfay and Noreen Goldman, "Reductions in 2020 U.S. Life Expectancy Due to COVID-19 and the Disproportionate Impact on the Black and Latino Populations," medRxiv, (October 2020), doi:10.1101/2020.07.12.20148387.

3. CDC, National Center for Health Statistics, "Life Expectancy in the U.S. Declined a Year and a Half in 2020," July 21, 2021, https://www.cdc.gov/nchs/pressroom/nchs_press_releases/2021/202107.htm.

CHAPTER 1

1. U.S. Census Bureau, "United States Population Projections: 2000 to 2050" (2018), https://www.census.gov/library/working-papers/2009/demo/us-pop-proj-2000-2050.html.

2. Elizabeth Arias and Jiquan Xu, "United States Life Tables," *National Vital Statistics Reports* 68, no. 7 (June 2019), https://www.cdc.gov/nchs/data/nvsr/nvsr68/nvsr68_07-508.pdf.

3. Max Roser, Esteban Ortiz-Ospina, and Hannah Ritchie, "Life Expectancy." *Our World in Data,* 2019, https://ourworldindata.org/life-expectancy.

4. Steven Woolf and Heidi Schoomaker, "Life Expectancy and Mortality Rates in the United States, 1959–2017," *JAMA* 322, no. 20 (2019): 1996–2016, doi:10.1001/jama.2019.16932.

5. Stein Emil Vollset, Emily Goren, Chun-Wei Yuan et al., "Fertility, Mortality, Migration, and Population Scenarios for 195 Countries and Territories From 2017 to 2100: A Forecasting Analysis for the Global Burden of Disease Study," *The Lancet* 396, no. 10258 (2020): 1285–1306, doi:10.1016/S0140-6736(20)30677-2.

6. Jeffrey S. Passel and D'Vera Cohn, "U.S. Population Projections: 2005–2050," Pew Research Center, 2008, https://www.pewresearch.org/hispanic/2008/02/11/us-population-projections-2005-2050.

7. Christopher Ingraham, "Look at How Much Weight You're Going to Gain," *Washington Post,* January 29, 2016, https://www.washingtonpost.com/news/wonk/wp/2016/01/29/the-age-when-you-gain-the-most-weight.

8. T. J. Sheehan, S. DuBrava, L. M. DeChello et al., "Rates of Weight Change for Black and White Americans Over a Twenty Year Period," *International Journal of Obesity* 27 no. 4 (2003): 498–504, doi:10.1038/sj.ijo.0802263.

9. JAMA Network Journals, "Weight Gain From Early to Middle Adulthood Linked to Increased Risk of Major Chronic Diseases, Death," *Eureka Alert,* July 18, 2017.

10. Nicholas S. Hendren, James A. de Lemos, Colby Ayers et al., "Association of Body Mass Index and Age With Morbidity and Mortality in Patients Hospitalized With COVID-19: Results From the American Heart Association COVID-19 Cardiovascular Disease Registry," *Circulation* 143 (2021): 135–144, doi:10.1161/CIRCULATIONAHA.120.051936.

11. Andrew J. Scott, Martin Ellison, and David A. Sinclair, "The Economic Value of Targeting Aging," *Nature Aging* 1 (2021): 616–623, doi: 10.1038/s43587-021-00080-0.

12. See *RealAge* and *YOU* books for a longer discussion of the importance of social connections to aging.

13. Gill Livingston, Andrew Sommerlad, Vasiliki Orgeta et al., "Dementia Prevention, Intervention, and Care," *The Lancet* 390, no. 10113 (2017): 2673–2734, doi:10.1016/S0140-6736(17)31363-6.

14. Harry Owen Taylor, Robert Joseph Taylor, Ann W. Nguyen et al., "Social Isolation, Depression,

and Psychological Distress Among Older Adults," *Journal of Aging and Health* 30, no. 2 (2018): 229–246, doi:10.1177/0898264316673511.

15. Isobel E. M. Evans, David J. Llewellyn, Fiona E. Matthews et al., "Social Isolation, Cognitive Reserve, and Cognition in Healthy Older People," *PLoS ONE* 13, no. 8 (2018): 1–14, doi:10.1371/ journal.pone.0201008.

CHAPTER 2

1. "System/360 Dates and Characteristics," IBM, https://www.ibm.com/ibm/history/exhibits /mainframe/mainframe_FS360.html; "Mainframe Computers," Computer History Museum, https://www.computerhistory.org/revolution/mainframe-computers/7/161–1965.

2. United Nations, Department of Economics and Social Affairs, *World Social Report 2020: Inequality in a Rapidly Changing World* (New York: United Nations, 2020).

PART 2
INTRODUCTION

1. Kirsten J. Colello and Angela Napili, "Older Americans Act: Overview and Funding," *Congressional Research Service* (April 22, 2021), https://crsreports.congress.gov/product/pdf/R/R43414.

2. "Too Many Patents," *Patent Progress* (2014). https://www.patentprogress.org/systemic-problems /too-many-patents.

3. Patrick Cox, *The Methuselah Effect—How the Trend Toward Longevity Is Accelerating—and Soon Will Turn Your World Upside Down* (Dallas: Mauldin Economics, 2016).

CHAPTER 3

1. Cleveland Clinic, "Heart Failure: Understanding Heart Failure," https://my.cleveland clinic.org/health/diseases/17069-heart-failure-understanding-heart-failure/management-and -treatment.

2. "Osaka University Transplants iPS Cell-Based Heart Cells in World's First Clinical Trial," *Japan Times,* January 28, 2020, https://www.japantimes.co.jp/news/2020/01/28/national/science -health/osaka-university-transplants-ips-cell-based-heart-cells-worlds-first-clinical-trial.

3. Satoshi Kainuma, Shigeru Miyagawa, Koichi Toda et al., "Long-Term Outcomes of Autologous Skeletal Myoblast Cell-Sheet Transplantation for End-Stage Ischemic Cardiomyopathy," *Molecular Therapy* 29, no. 4 (April 2021), doi: 10.1016/j.ymthe.2021.01.004.

4. "Neurons at the Laboratory Can Be Integrated Into Human Brain Tissue," Universitat de Barcelona, August 27, 2020, https://www.ub.edu/web/ub/en/menu_eines/noticies/2020/08/004.html.

5. Beatriz Suárez-Álvarez, Ramón M. Rodriguez, Vincenzo Calvanese et al., "Epigenetic Mechanisms Regulate MHC and Antigen Processing Molecules in Human Embryonic and Induced Pluripotent Stem Cells," *PLoS ONE* 5, no. 4 (2010): e10192. doi.org/10.1371/journal.pone.0010192.

6. Ratnesh Singh, Oscar Cuzzani, François Binette et al., "Pluripotent Stem Cells for Retinal Tissue Engineering: Current Status and Future Prospects," *Stem Cell Reviews and Reports* 14, no. 4 (2018): 463–483, doi:10.1007/s12015-018-9802-4.

7. Federico Quaini, Konrad Urbanek, Antonio P. Beltrami et al., "Chimerism of the Transplanted Heart," *New England Journal of Medicine* 346, no. 1 (2002): 5–15.

8. Jerry W. Shay and Woodring E. Wright, "Hayflick, His Limit, and Cellular Ageing," *Nature Reviews Molecular Cell Biology* 1 (2000): 72–76, doi:10.1038/35036093.

9. Yafit Hachmo, Amir Hadanny, Ramzia Abu Hamed et al., "Hyperbaric Oxygen Therapy Increases Telomere Length and Decreases Immunosenescence in Isolated Blood Cells: A Prospective Trial," *Aging* 12, no. 22 (2020): 22445–22456, doi:10.18632/aging.202188.

10. Joy Q. He, Eric S. Sussman, and Gary K. Steinberg, "Revisiting Stem Cell-Based Clinical Trials for Ischemic Stroke," *Frontiers in Aging Neuroscience* 12 (December 14, 2020): 575990, doi:10.3389/fnagi.2020.575990.

11. Charles A. Goldthwaite, Jr., "The Promise of Induced Pluripotent Stem Cells (iPSCs)," in *Regenerative Medicine* (Bethesda, Md: National Institutes of Health, 2006).

12. Changhan Lee and Valter Longo, "Dietary Restriction With and Without Caloric Restriction for Healthy Aging," *F1000Research* 5 (January 29, 2016): 117, doi:10.12688/f1000research.7136.1.

13. Rafael de Cabo and Mark P. Mattson, "Effects of Intermittent Fasting on Health, Aging, and Disease," *New England Journal of Medicine* 381 (2019): 2541–2551.

14. Hyung Wook Park, "Longevity, Aging, and Caloric Restriction: Clive Maine McCay and the Construction of a Multidisciplinary Research Program," *Natural Sciences* 40, no. 1 (Winter 2010): 79–124, doi:10.1525/hsns.2010.40.1.79.

15. Wen-Chung Tsai, Tung-Yang Yu, Gwo-Jyh Chang et al., "Platelet-Rich Plasma Releasate Promotes Regeneration and Decreases Inflammation and Apoptosis of Injured Skeletal Muscle," *American Journal of Sports Medicine* 46, no. 8 (2018): 198–1986, doi:10.1177/0363546518771076.

16. Karthik Arumugam, William Shin, Valentina Schiavone et al., "The Master Regulator Protein BAZ2B Can Reprogram Human Hematopoietic Lineage-Committed Progenitors Into a Multipotent State," *Cell Reports* 33, no. 10 (December 8, 2020): 108474, doi:10.1016/j.celrep.2020.10847.

CHAPTER 4

1. Tamara Tchkonia, Yi Zhu, Jan van Deursen et al., "Cellular Senescence and the Senescent Secretory Phenotype: Therapeutic Opportunities," *Journal of Clinical Investigation* 123, no. 3 (2013): 966–972, doi:10.1172/JCI64098. See also: Susan Buckles, "Turning the Clock Back on Aging," Mayo Clinic Center for Regenerative Medicine, September 17, 2020, https://regenerativemedicineblog.mayoclinic.org/2020/09/17/turning-the-clock-back-on-aging/.

2. UNITY Biotechnology, "UNITY Biotechnology Announces 12-Week Data From UBX0101 Phase 2 Clinical Study in Patients With Painful Osteoarthritis of the Knee," *GlobeNewswire*, August 17, 2020.

3. Saul A. Villeda, Kristopher E. Plambeck, Jinte Middeldorp et al., "Young Blood Reverses Age-Related Impairments in Cognitive Function and Synaptic Plasticity in Mice," *Nature Medicine* 20 (2014): 659–663, doi: 10.1038/nm.3569.

4. Judith Campisi, Pankaj Kapahi, Gordon J. Lithgow et al., "From Discoveries in Ageing Research to Therapeutics for Healthy Ageing," *Nature* 571, no. 7764 (2019): 183–192.

5. Steve Horvath, Kavita Singh, Ken Raj et al., "Reversing Age: Dual Species Measurement of Epigenetic Age With a Single Clock," *bioRxiv* (2020), doi:10.1101/2020.05.07.082917.

6. Keng Siang Lee, Shuxiao Lin, David A. Copland et al., "Cellular Senescence in the Aging Retina and Developments of Senotherapies for Age-Related Macular Degeneration," *Journal of Neuroinflammation* 18, no. 32 (2021), doi:10.1186/s12974-021-02088-0.

7. Louisa Chou, Tom A. Ranger, Waruna Peiris et al., "Patients' Perceived Needs for Medical Services for Non-Specific Low Back Pain: A Systematic Scoping Review," *PLoS One* 13, no. 11 (2018), doi:10.1371/journal.pone.0204885.

8. Brian Gehlbach and Eugene Geppert, "The Pulmonary Manifestations of Left Heart Failure," *Chest* 125 (2004): 669–682.

9. J. L. Kirkland and T. Tchkonia, "Senolytic Drugs: From Discovery to Translation," *Journal of Internal Medicine* 288, no. 5 (November 2020): 518–536, doi:10.1111/joim.13141.

10. Anna Walaszczyk, Emily Dookun, Rachael Redgrave et al., "Pharmacological Clearance of Senescent Cells Improves Survival and Recovery in Aged Mice Following Acute Myocardial Infarction," *Aging Cell* 18, no. 3 (2019): e12945.

11. Sarbari Saha, Debasna P. Panigrahi, Shankargouda Patil et al., "Autophagy in Health and Disease: A Comprehensive Review," *Biomedicine & Pharmacotherapy* 104 (2018): 485–495.

12. Mohammad Bagherniya, Alexandra E. Butler, George E. Barreto et al., "The Effect of Fasting or Calorie Restriction on Autophagy Induction: A Review of the Literature," *Ageing Research Reviews* 47 (2018): 183–197, doi:10.1016/j.arr.2018.08.004.

13. Laura Poillet-Perez and Eileen White, "Role of Tumor and Host Autophagy in Cancer Metabolism," *Genes & Development* 33 (2019): 610–619, doi:10.1101/gad.325514.119.

14. Laura Poillet-Perez, Xiaoqi Xie, Le Zhan et al., "Autophagy Maintains Tumour Growth Through Circulating Arginine," *Nature* 563 (2018): 569–573, doi:10.1038/s41586-018-0697-7.

15. Melod Mehdipour, Colin Skinner, Nathan Wong et al., "Rejuvenation of Three Germ Layers Tissues by Exchanging Old Blood Plasma With Saline-Albumin," *Aging* 12, no. 10 (2020): 8790–8819, doi:10.18632/aging.103418.

16. David A. Sinclair and Matthew D. LaPlante, *Lifespan: Why We Age—and Why We Don't Have To* (New York: Thorsons, 2019).

CHAPTER 5

1. Zhongqiu Xie, Pawel Ł. Janczyk, Yingg Zhang et al., "A Cytoskeleton Regulator AVIL Drives Tumorigenesis in Glioblastoma," *Nature Communications* 11, article no. 3457 (2020), doi:10.1038/s41467-020-17279-1.

2. The American Association for Cancer Research Human Epigenome Task Force and European Union, Network of Excellence, Scientific Advisory Board, "Moving AHEAD With an International Human Epigenome Project," *Nature* 454 (2008): 711–715, doi:10.1038/454711a.

3. Elissa S. Epel, Elizabeth H. Blackburn, Jue Lin et al., "Accelerated Telomere Shortening in Response to Life Stress," *Proceedings of the National Academy of Sciences* 101, no. 49 (December 2004): 17312–17315, doi:10.1073/pnas.0407162101.

4. Dean Ornish, Mark Jesus M. Magbanua, Gerdi Weidner et al., "Changes in Prostate Gene Expression in Men Undergoing an Intensive Nutrition and Lifestyle Intervention." *Proceedings of the National Academy of Sciences* 105, no. 24 (June 2008): 8369–8374, doi:10.1073/pnas.0803080105.

5. Francisco Martínez-Jiménez, Ferran Muiños, Inés Sentís et al., "A Compendium of Mutational Cancer Driver Genes," *Nature Reviews Cancer* 20 (2020): 555–572, doi:10.1038/s41568-020-0290-x.

6. Apresio K. Fajrial, Qing Qing He, Nurul I. Wirusanti et al., "A Review of Emerging Physical Transfection Methods for CRISPR/Cas9-Mediated Gene Editing," *Theranostics* 10, no. 12 (2020): 5532–5549.

7. Shao-Shuai Wu, Qing-Cui Li, Chang-Qing Yin et al., "Advances in CRISPR/Cas-based Gene Therapy in Human Genetic Diseases," *Theranostics* 10, no. 10 (2020): 4374–4382, doi:10.7150/thno.43360.

8. Vera Lucia Raposo, "The First Chinese Edited Babies: A Leap of Faith in Science," *JBRA Assisted Reproduction* 23, no. 3 (2019): 197–199, doi:10.5935/1518-0557.20190042.

9. Haydar Frangoul, David Altshuler, M. Domenica Cappellini et al., "CRISPR-Cas9 Gene Editing for Sickle Cell Disease and β-Thalassemia," *New England Journal of Medicine* 384 (2021): 252–260, doi:10.1056/NEJMoa2031054.

10. Eliot Marshall, "Gene Therapy Death Prompts Review of Adenovirus Vector," *Science* 286, no. 5448 (December 17, 1999): 2244–2245.

11. Alejandro Ocampo, Pradeep Reddy, Paloma Martinez-Redondo et al., "In Vivo Amelioration of Age-Associated Hallmarks by Partial Reprogramming," *Cell* 167, no. 7 (December 15, 2016): 1719–1733.E12, doi:10.1016/j.cell.2016.11.052.

12. Antonio Regalado, "A Stealthy Harvard Startup Wants to Reverse Aging in Dogs, and Humans Could Be Next," *MIT Technology Review,* May 9, 2018.

13. Shinya Yamanaka, "Induced Pluripotent Stem Cells: Past, Present, and Future," *Cell Stem Cell* 10, no. 6 (June 14, 2012): 678–684.

14. Jeremy Michael Van Raamsdonk, and Siegfried Hekimi, "FUdR Causes a Twofold Increase in the Lifespan of the Mitochondrial Mutant gas-1," *Mechanisms of Ageing and Development* 132, no. 10 (2011): 519–521.

15. Yuancheng Lu, Benedikt Brommer, Xiao Tian et al., "Reprogramming to Recover Youthful Epigenetic Information and Restore Vision," *Nature* 588 (2020): 124–129, doi:10.1038/s41586-020-2975-4.

16. George M. Martin, Steven N. Austad, and Thomas E. Johnson, "Genetic Analysis of Ageing: Role of Oxidative Damage and Environmental Stresses," *Nature Genetics* 13, no. 1 (May 1996): 25–34.

17. Jianfeng Lan, Jarod A. Rollins, Xiao Zang et al., "Translational Regulation of Non-autonomous Mitochondrial Stress Response Promotes Longevity," *Cell Reports* 28, no. 4 (2019): 1050–1062.e6, doi: 10.1016/j.celrep.2019.06.078.

18. Giacamo Cavalli and Edith Heard, "Advances in Epigenetics Link Genetics to the Environment and Disease," *Nature* 571 (2019): 489–499, doi:10.1038/s41586-019-1411-0.

19. Mohamed M. Ali, Dina Naquiallah, Maryam Qureshi et al., "DNA Methylation Profile of Genes Involved in Inflammation and Autoimmunity Correlates With Vascular Function in Morbidly Obese Adults," *Epigenetics* (2021), doi:10.1080/15592294.2021.1876285.

20. David A. Sinclair and Matthew D. LaPlante, *Lifespan: Why We Age—and Why We Don't Have To* (New York: Thorsons, 2019).

21. RMIT University, "Metal-Organic Frameworks Successfully Deliver CRISPR/Cas9 Into Human Cancer Cells," *Technology Networks,* November 23, 2020.

22. Redouane Aherrahrou, Liang Guo, V. Peter Nagraj et al., "Genetic Regulation of Atherosclerosis-Relevant Phenotypes in Human Vascular Smooth Muscle Cells," *Circulation Research* 127 (2020): 1552–1565, doi:10.1161/CIRCRESAHA.120.317415.

CHAPTER 6

1. K. Esfahani, L. Roudaia, N. Buhlaiga et al., "A Review of Cancer Immunotherapy: From the Past, to the Present, to the Future," *Current Oncology* 27, suppl. 2 (2020) 87–97, doi:10.3747/co.27.5223.

2. Charles N. Serhan and Bruce D. Levy, "Resolvins in Inflammation: Emergence of the Pro-Resolving Superfamily of Mediators," *Journal of Clinical Investigation* 128, no. 7 (2018): 2657–2669, doi:10.1172/JCI97943.

3. Sara Campinoti, Asllan Gjinovci, Roberta Ragazzini et al., "Reconstitution of a Functional Human Thymus by Postnatal Stromal Progenitor Cells and Natural Whole-Organ Scaffolds," *Nature Communications* 11, article no. 6372 (2020), doi:10.1038/s41467-020-20082-7.

4. Jeffrey A. Haspel, Ron Anafi, Marishka K. Brown et al., "Perfect Timing: Circadian Rhythms, Sleep, and Immunity—An NIH Workshop Summary," *JCI Insight* 5, no. 1 (January 16, 2020): e131487, doi:10.1172/jci.insight.131487.

5. Adrian F. Gombart, Adeline Pierre, and Silvia Maggini, "A Review of Micronutrients and the Immune System–Working in Harmony to Reduce the Risk of Infection," *Nutrients* 12, no. 1 (2020): 236, doi:10.3390/nu12010236.

6. Michael F. Roizen and Michael C. Crupain, *What to Eat When: A Strategic Plan to Improve Your Health & Life Through Food* (Washington, D.C.: National Geographic, 2019).

7. James P. Allison, "Immune Checkpoint Blockade in Cancer Therapy: The 2015 Lasker-DeBakey Clinical Medical Research Award," *JAMA* 314, no. 11 (2015): 1113–1114, and personal communication with J. P. Allison.

8. Michael J. Eppihimer, Jason Gunn, Gordon J. et al., "Expression and Regulation of the PD-L1 Immunoinhibitory Molecule on Microvascular Endothelial Cells," *Microcirculation* 9, no. , 133–145, doi: 10.1038/sj/mn/7800123.

9. Philip C. Calder, "Nutrition, Immunity and COVID-19," BMJ *Nutrition, Prevention & Health* 3, no. 1 (2020), doi:10.1136/bmjnph-2020-000085.

10. Hasan Ejaz, Abdullah Alsrhani, Aizza Zafar et al., "COVID-19 and Comorbidities: Deleterious Impact on Infected Patients," *Journal of Infection and Public Health* 13, no. 12 (December 12, 2020): 1833–1839, doi:10.1016/j.jiph.2020.07.014.

11. Robert J. Mason, "Pathogenesis of COVID-19 From a Cell Biology Perspective," *European Respiratory Journal* 55, no. 4 (April 2020): 2000607, doi:10.1183/13993003.00607-2020.

12. Centers for Disease Control and Prevention, "Understanding How Vaccines Work," https://www.cdc .gov/vaccines/hcp/conversations/understanding-vacc-work.html (accessed November 28, 2021).

13. David M. Margolis, Richard A. Koup, and Guido Ferrari, "HIV Antibodies for Treatment of HIV Infection," *Immunological Reviews* 275, no. 1 (2017): 313–323, doi:10.1111/imr.12506.

14. Steve Black, David E. Bloom, David C. Kaslow et al., "Transforming Vaccine Development," *Seminars in Immunology* 50 (August 2020): 101413, doi:10.1016/j.smim.2020.101413.

15. Luca Vangelista and Massimiliano Secchi, "Prepare for the Future: Dissecting the Spike to Seek Broadly Neutralizing Antibodies and Universal Vaccine for Pandemic Coronaviruses," *Frontiers in Molecular Biosciences* 7 (September 1, 2020): 226, doi:10.3389/fmolb.2020.00226.

16. Nir Eyal, Marc Lipsitch, and Peter G. Smith, "Human Challenge Studies to Accelerate Coronavirus Vaccine Licensure," *Journal of Infectious Diseases* 221, no. 11 (June 1, 2020): 1752–1756, doi:10.1093/infdis/jiaa152.

17. Viveksandeep Thoguluva Chandrasekar, Bhanuprasad Vankatesalu, Harsh K. Patel et al., "Systematic Review and Meta-Analysis of Effectiveness of Treatment Options Against SARS-CoV-2 Infection," *Journal of Medical Virology* 93, no. 2 (2021): 775–785. doi:10.1002/jmv.26302.

18. Xueqing Wang and Yuanfang Guan, "COVID-19 Drug Repurposing: A Review of Computational Screening Methods, Clinical Trials, and Protein Interaction Assays," *Medicinal Research Reviews* 41, no. 1 (2021): 5–28, doi:10.1002/med.21728.

19. Juanita Mellet and Michael S. Pepper, "A COVID-19 Vaccine: Big Strides Come With Big Challenges," *Vaccines* 9, no. 1 (2021): 39, doi:10.3390/vaccines9010039.

CHAPTER 7

1. Denis P. Blondin, Soren Nielsen, Eline N. Kuipers et al., "Human Brown Adipocyte Thermogenesis Is Driven by β2-AR Stimulation," *Cell Metabolism* 32, no. 2 (August 4, 2020): 287–300. E7, doi:10.1016/j.cmet.2020.07.005.

2. Centers for Disease Control and Prevention, "Adult Obesity Facts," https://www.cdc.gov/obesity/data/adult.html (accessed February 16, 2021).

3. Ying-Xin Shi, Xiang-Yu Chen, Hui-Na Qiu et al., "Visceral Fat Area to Appendicular Muscle Mass Ratio as a Predictor for Nonalcoholic Fatty Liver Disease Independent of Obesity," *Scandinavian Journal of Gastroenterology* (2021), doi:10.1080/00365521.2021.1879244.

4. Tobias Becher, Srikanth Palanisamy, Daniel J. Kramer et al., "Brown Adipose Tissue Is Associated With Cardiometabolic Health," *Nature Medicine* 27 (2021): 58–65, doi:10.1038/s41591-020-1126-7.

5. Yanhong Shi, Haruhisa Inoue, Joseph C. Wu et al., "Induced Pluripotent Stem Cell Technology: A Decade of Progress," *Nature Reviews Drug Discovery* 16 (2017): 115–130, doi:10.1038/nrd.2016.245.

6. Michael West, Dana Larocca, and Jieun Lee, "Induced Tissue Regeneration Using Extracellular Vesicles," U.S. Patent App. 16/833285, https://uspto.report/patent/app/20200306296 (accessed February 16, 2021).

7. Alice Rossi, Paola Pizzo, and Riccardo Filadi, "Calcium, Mitochondria and Cell Metabolism: A Functional Triangle in Bioenergetics," *Biochimica et Biophysica Acta (BBA)—Molecular Cell Research* 1866, no. 7 (2019): 1068–1078, doi:10.1016/j.bbamcr.2018.10.016.

8. I. Sánchez-González, A. Jiménez-Escrig, and F. Saura-Calixto, "In Vitro Antioxidant Activity of Coffees Brewed Using Different Procedures (Italian, Espresso and Filter)," *Food Chemistry* 90, nos. 1–2, (2005): 133–139.

9. Jianmei Zhang, Huixiao Wu, Shizhan Ma et al., "Transcription Regulators and Hormones Involved in the Development of Brown Fat and White Fat Browning: Transcriptional and Hormonal Control of Brown/Beige Fat Development," *Physiological Research* 67, no. 3 (2018): 347–362.

10. Michael D. West, Ching-Fang Chang, Dana Larocca et al., "Clonal Derivation of White and Brown Adipocyte Progenitor Cell Lines From Human Pluripotent Stem Cells," *Stem Cell Research & Therapy* 10 (2019): 1–17.

11. Mathieu Panel, Bijan Ghaleh, and Didier Morin, "Mitochondria and Aging: A Role for the Mitochondrial Transition Pore?" *Aging Cell* 17, no. 4 (2018): e12793, doi:10.1111/acel.12793.

12. Xian Xie, Yi Gao, Min Zeng et al., "Nicotinamide Ribose Ameliorates Cognitive Impairment of Aged and Alzheimer's Disease Model Mice," *Metabolic Brain Disease* 34, no. 1 (2019): 353–366.

CHAPTER 8

1. Alyssa M. Flores, Niloufar Hosseini-Nassab, Kai-Uwe Jarr et al., "Pro-Efferocytic Nanoparticles Are Specifically Taken Up by Lesional Macrophages and Prevent Atherosclerosis," *Nature Nanotechnology* 15 (2020): 154–161, doi:10.1038/s41565-019-0619-3.

2. Catherine Saint Louis, "Doctors Experiment With New Way of Fixing the A.C.L.," *New York Times*, March 23, 2016.

3. Bagrat Grigoryan, Samantha J. Paulsen, Daniel C. Corbett et al., "Multivascular Networks and Functional Intravascular Topologies Within Biocompatible Hydrogels," *Science* 364, no. 6439 (2019): 458–464. doi:10.1126/science.aav9750.

4. Tamra Sami, "Aussie Startup Inventia Could Revolutionize Skin Regeneration With 3D Bioprinting Robot," *BioWorld*, July 31, 2020.

5. Sangsoon Park, Murat Artan, Seung Hyun Han et al., "VRK-1 Extends Life Span by Activation of AMPK Via Phosphorylation," *Science Advances* 6, no. 27 (2020): eaaw7824, doi:10.1126/sciadv.aaw7824.

6. Mark F. Newman, Joseph P. Mathew, Hilary P. Grocott et al., "Central Nervous System Injury Associated With Cardiac Surgery," *The Lancet* 368, no. 9536 (2006): 694–703, doi:10.1016/S0140-6736(06)69254-4.

7. Augusto D'Onofrio and Gino Gerosa, "Shifting a Paradigm of Cardiac Surgery: From Minimally Invasive to Micro-Invasive," *Journal of Heart Valve Disease* 24, no. 5 (September 2015): 528–530.

8. C. C. J. Alcântara, F. C. Landers, S. Kim et al., "Mechanically Interlocked 3D Multi-Material Micromachines," *Nature Communications* 11, no. 5957 (2020), doi:10.1038/s41467-020-19725-6.

9. Abby Roth, "New Global Ultrasound POCUS Is No Hocus," *Yale Medicine* (Summer 2019).

10. Thomas Franck, "Human Lifespan Could Soon Pass 100 Years Thanks to Medical Tech, Says BofA," CNBC.com, May 8, 2019.

PART 3
CHAPTER 9

1. Harriet Edleson, "Almost Half of Americans Fear Running Out of Money in Retirement," AARP, May 21, 2019.

2. Steven H. Woolf and Heidi Schoomaker, "Life Expectancy and Mortality Rates in the United States, 1959–2017," *JAMA* 322, no. 20 (2019): 1996–2016, doi:10.1001/jama.2019.16932.

3. U.S. Census Bureau, 2017 National Population Projection Tables, Table 1: Projected Population

Size and Births, Deaths, and Migration, https://www.census.gov/data/tables/2017/demo/popproj/2017-summary-tables.html (accessed February 17, 2021).

4. John A. Jagerson and Margaret James, "What Is the Formula for Calculating Net Present Value (NPV)?" Investopedia, January 16, 2021, https://www.investopedia.com/ask/answers/032615/what-formula-calculating-net-present-value-npv.asp (accessed February 17, 2021).

5. Andrew J. Scott, Martin Ellison, and David A. Sinclair, "The Economic Value of Targeting Aging," *Nature Aging* 1 (2021): 616–623, doi: 10.1038/s43587-021-00080-0.

6. U.S. Bureau of Labor Statistics, Monthly Labor Review, "Labor Force Projections to 2022: The Labor Force Participation Rate Continues to Fall," https://www.bls.gov/opub/mlr/2013/article/labor-force-projections-to-2022-the-labor-force-participation-rate-continues-to-fall.htm (accessed February 17, 2021).

7. Melissa A. Z. Knoll, "Behavioral and Psychological Aspects of the Retirement Decision," *Social Security Bulletin* 71, no. 4 (2011), https://www.ssa.gov/policy/docs/ssb/v71n4/v71n4p15.html (accessed February 17, 2021).

8. Centers for Disease Control and Prevention, "Health and Economic Costs of Chronic Diseases," https://www.cdc.gov/chronicdisease/about/costs/index.htm (accessed February 17, 2021).

9. The Week Staff, "The Inheritance Boom," *The Week*, December 7, 2019.

CHAPTER 10

1. Lilah M. Besser, Merilee A. Teylan, and Peter T. Nelson, "Limbic Predominant Age-Related TDP-43 Encephalopathy (LATE): Clinical and Neuropathological Associations." *Journal of Neuropathology & Experimental Neurology* 79, no. 3 (2020): 305–313, doi:10.1093/jnen/nlz126.

2. Jennaya Christensen, Glenn R. Yamakawa, Sandy R. Shultz et al., "Is the Glymphatic System the Missing Link Between Sleep Impairments and Neurological Disorders? Examining the Implications and Uncertainties," *Progress in Neurobiology* 198 (2020): 101917, doi:10.1016/j.pneurobio.2020.101917.

3. Natalie L. Hauglund, Chiara Pavan, and Maiken Nedergaard, "Cleaning the Sleeping Brain—The Potential Restorative Function of the Glymphatic System," *Current Opinion in Physiology* 15 (2020): 1–6, doi:10.1016/j.cophys.2019.10.020.

4. Nicola L. Francis, Nanxia Zhao, Hannah R. Calvelli et al., "Peptide-Based Scaffolds for the Culture and Transplantation of Human Dopaminergic Neurons." *Tissue Engineering Part A* 26, nos. 3–4 (2020): 193–205, doi:10.1089/ten.tea.2019.0094.

5. Mercè Boada, Oscar L. López, Javier Olazarán et al., "Neurophysiological , Neuropsychiatric, and Quality-of-Life Assessments in Alzheimer's Disease Patients Treated With Plasma Exchange With Albumin Replacement From the Randomized AMBAR Study," *Alzheimer's & Dementia* 17 (2021): 1–11, doi:10.1002/alz.12477.

6. Eva Ausó, Violeta Gómez-Vicente, and Gema Esquiva, "Biomarkers for Alzheimer's Disease Early Diagnosis," *Journal of Personalized Medicine* 10, no. 3 (2020): 114, doi:10.3390/jpm10030114.

7. Jessica Mozersky, Sarah Hartz, Erin Linnenbringer et al., "Communicating 5-Year Risk of

Sources

Alzheimer's Disease Dementia: Development and Evaluation of Materials That Incorporate Multiple Genetic and Biomarker Research Results." *Journal of Alzheimer's Disease* 79, no. 2 (2021): 559–572, doi:10.3233/JAD-200993.

8. Aaron Arvey, Michael Rowe, Joseph Barten Legutki et al., "Age-Associated Changes in the Circulating Human Antibody Repertoire Are Upregulated in Autoimmunity," *Immunity & Ageing* 17 (2020), doi:10.1186/s12979-020-00193-x.

9. Rachel Thomas, Weikan Wang, and Dong-Ming Su, "Contributions of Age-Related Thymic Involution to Immunosenescence and Inflammaging," *Immunity & Ageing* 17 (2020), doi:10.1186/s12979-020-0173-8.

10. Jamal S. Rana, Sadiya S. Khan, Donald M. Lloyd-Jones et al., "Changes in Mortality in Top 10 Causes of Death From 2011 to 2018," *Journal of General Internal Medicine* (2020), doi:10.1007/s11606-020-06070-z.

11. Walter Kempner, "Treatment of Heart and Kidney Disease and of Hypertensive and Arteriosclerotic Vascular Disease With the Rice Diet," *Annals of Internal Medicine* 31, no. 5 (1949): 821–856, doi:10.7326/0003-4819-31-5-821.

12. Andrew M. Freeman, Pamela B. Morris, Neal Barnard et al., "Trending Cardiovascular Nutrition Controversies," *Journal of the American College of Cardiology* 69, no. 9 (2017): 1172–1187, doi:10.1016/j.jacc.2016.10.086.

13. Paul K. Whelton and Robert M. Carey, "The 2017 Clinical Practice Guideline for High Blood Pressure," *JAMA* 318, no. 21 (2017): 2073–2074, doi:10.1001/jama.2017.18209.

14. F. M. Sones Jr. and E. K. Shirey, "Cine Coronary Arteriography," *Modern Concepts of Cardiovascular Disease* 31 (1962): 735–738.

15. F. Nijland, O. Kamp, P. M. J. Verhorst et al., "Early Prediction of Improvement in Ejection Fraction After Acute Myocardial Infarction Using Low Dose Dobutamine Echocardiography," *Heart* 88, no. 6 (2002): 592–596, doi:10.1136/heart.88.6.592.

16. Cleveland Clinic, "Why Diastolic Dysfunction Raises Death Risk," https://health.clevelandclinic.org/death-risk-for-diastolic-dysfunction (accessed February 21, 2021).

17. Leonardo Bandeira, E. Michael Lewiecki, and John P. Bilezikian, "Romosozumab for the Treatment of Osteoporosis," *Expert Opinion on Biological Therapy* 17, no. 2 (2017): 255–263, doi:10.1080/14712598.2017.1280455.

18. Catherine Saint Louis, "Doctors Experiment With New Way of Fixing the A.C.L.," *New York Times*, March 23, 2016.

19. Yuancheng Lu, Anitha Krishnan, Benedikt Brommer et al., "Reversal of Ageing- and Injury-Induced Vision Loss by Tet-Dependent Epigenetic Reprogramming," *bioRxiv* (2019), doi:10.1101/710210.

20. Jussi J. Paterno, Ali Koskela, Juha M. T. Hyttinen et al., "Autophagy Genes for Wet Age-Related Macular Degeneration in a Finnish Case-Control Study," *Genes* 11, no. 11 (2020): 1318, doi:10.3390/genes11111318.

21. Keng Siang Lee, Shuxiao Lin, David A. Copland et al., "Cellular Senescence in the Aging Retina and Developments of Senotherapies for Age-Related Macular Degeneration," *Journal of Neuroinflammation* 18, article no. 32 (2021), doi:10.1186/s12974-021-02088-0.

22. Arianna Di Stadio, Massimo Ralli, Dalila Roccamatisi et al., "Hearing Loss and Dementia: Radiologic

and Biomolecular Basis of Their Shared Characteristics. A Systematic Review," *Neurological Sciences* 42 (2021): 579–588, doi.org/10.1007/s10072-020-04948-8.

23. Frank R. Lin, Kristine Yaffe, Jin Xia et al., "Hearing Loss and Cognitive Decline in Older Adults," *JAMA Internal Medicine* 173, no. 4 (2013): 293–299, doi:10.1001/jamainternmed.2013.1868.

PART 4
CHAPTER 11

1. David E. Newman-Toker, Adam C. Schaffer, C. Winnie Yu-Moe et al., "Serious Misdiagnosis-Related Harms in Malpractice Claims: The 'Big Three'—Vascular Events, Infections, and Cancers," *Diagnosis* 6, no. 3 (2019): 227–240, doi: 10.1515/dx-2019-0019.

2. Michael F. Roizen and Mehmet C. Oz, *YOU: The Smart Patient. An Insider's Handbook for Getting the Best Treatment* (New York: Scribner, 2006).

3. K. W. Jamieson, *A World in Two Minds: Why We Must Change Our Thinking to Change Our Future* (Edinburgh: Shepheard-Walwyn, 2020).

4. Chris Charyk, "The Pros and Cons of Pros-and-Cons Lists," *Harvard Business Review* (January 6, 2017).

5. Erick Larson, "A Checklist for Making Faster, Better Decisions," *Harvard Business Review* (March 7, 2016).

6. Nadav Even Chorev, "Personalized Medicine in Practice: Postgenomics From Multiplicity to Immutability," *Body & Society* 26, no. 1 (2020): 26–54, doi:10.1177/1357034X19886925.

CHAPTER 12

1. Dean Ornish, Mark Jesus M. Magbanua, Gerdi Weidner et al., "Changes in Prostate Gene Expression in Men Undergoing an Intensive Nutrition and Lifestyle Intervention," *Proceedings of the National Academy of Sciences* 105, no. 24 (2008): 8369–8374, doi:10.1073/pnas .0803080105.

2. Kaare Christensen, Niels V. Holm, Matt Mcgue et al., "A Danish Population-Based Twin Study on General Health in the Elderly," *Journal of Aging and Health* 11, no. 1 (February 1999): 49–64, doi.org/10.1177/089826439901100103.

3. Michael F. Roizen, *RealAge: Are You as Young as You Can Be?* (New York: Harper Collins, 1999).

4. Prateek Lohia, Shweta Kapur, Sindhuri Benjaram et al., "Metabolic Syndrome and Clinical Outcomes in Patients Infected With COVID-19: Does Age, Sex, and Race of the Patient With Metabolic Syndrome Matter?" *Journal of Diabetes* (2021), doi.org/10.1111/1753 -0407.13157.

5. Terrance L. Albrecht and Mara B. Adelman, "Social Support and Life Stress: New Directions for Communication Research," *Human Communication Research* 11, no. 1 (1984): 3–32, doi:10.1111/j.1468-2958.1984.tb00036.x

6. Nell H. Gottlieb and Lawrence W. Green, "Life Events, Social Network, Life-Style, and Health: An Analysis of the 1979 National Survey of Personal Health Practices and Consequences," *Health Education & Behavior* 11, issue 1 (1984): 91–105, doi:10.1177/109019818401100105.

7. Michael F. Roizen, *RealAge Makeover: Take Years Off Your Looks and Add Them to Your Life* (New York: Harper Collins, 2004).

8. Klodian Dhana, Denis A. Evans, Kumar B. Rajan et al., "Healthy Lifestyle and the Risk of Alzheimer Dementia: Findings From 2 Longitudinal Studies," *Neurology* 95, no. 4 (2020): e374–e383, doi:10.1212/WNL.0000000000009816.

9. Michael F. Roizen, *This Is Your Do-Over: The 7 Secrets to Losing Weight, Living Longer, and Getting a Second Chance at the Life You Want* (New York: Scribner, 2016).

10. Personal communication with CEO of EXOS.

CHAPTER 13

1. Didier Allexandre, Adam M. Bernstein, Esteban Walker et al., "A Web-Based Mindfulness Stress Management Program in a Corporate Call Center: A Randomized Clinical Trial to Evaluate the Added Benefit of Onsite Group Support," *Journal of Occupational and Environmental Medicine* 58, no. 3 (March 2016): 254–264, doi:10.1097/JOM.0000000000000680.

2. Jean Chatzky and Michael F. Roizen, *Age Proof: Living Longer Without Running Out of Money or Breaking a Hip* (New York: Grand Central Publishing, 2017).

3. Tavia E. Evans, Hieab H. H. Adams, Silvan Licher et al., "Subregional Volumes of the Hippocampus in Relation to Cognitive Function and Risk of Dementia," *Neuroimage* 178 (September 2018): 129–135, doi:10.1016/j.neuroimage.2018.05.041.

4. Juga Lee, "The Relationship Between Physical Activity and Dementia: A Systematic Review and Meta-Analysis of Prospective Cohort Studies," *Journal of Gerontological Nursing* 44, no. 10 (2018): 22–29, doi:10.3928/00989134-20180814-01.

5. Gill Livingston, Andrew Sommerlad, Vasiliki Orgeta et al., "Dementia Prevention, Intervention, and Care," *The Lancet* 390, no. 10113 (2017): 2673–2734, doi:10.1016/S0140-6736(17)31363-6.

6. Natan Feter, Gregore I. Mielke, Jayne S. Leite et al., "Physical Activity in Later Life and Risk of Dementia: Findings From a Population-Based Cohort Study," *Experimental Gerontology* 143 (2021): 111145, doi:10.1016/j.exger.2020.111145.

7. Aishat T. Bakre, Ruoling Chen, Ranjit Khutan et al., "Association Between Fish Consumption and Risk of Dementia: A New Study From China and a Systematic Literature Review and Meta-Analysis," *Public Health Nutrition* 21, no. 10 (2018): 1921–1932, doi:10.1017/S136898001800037X.

8. Karin Yurko-Mauro, Deanna McCarthy, Dror Rom et al., "Beneficial Effects of Docosahexaenoic Acid on Cognition in Age-Related Cognitive Decline." *Alzheimer's & Dementia* 6, no. 6 (2010): 456–464, doi:10.1016/j.jalz.2010.01.013.

9. Yang Hu, Frank B. Hu, and JoAnn E. Manson,"Marine Omega-3 Supplementation and Cardiovascular Disease: An Updated Meta-Analysis of 13 Randomized Controlled Trials Involving 127 477 Participants," *Journal of the American Heart Association* 8, no. 19 (2019): e013543, doi:10.1161/JAHA.119.013543.

10. Aldo A. Bernasconi, Michelle M. Wiest, Carl J. Lavie et al., "Effect of Omega-3 Dosage on Cardiovascular Outcomes," *Mayo Clinic Proceedings* 96, no. 2 (2021): 304–31, doi:10.1016/j.mayocp.2020.08.034.

11. Neal D. Barnard, Jihad Alwarith, Emilie Rembert et al., "A Mediterranean Diet and Low-Fat Vegan Diet to Improve Body Weight and Cardiometabolic Risk Factors: A Randomized, Cross-over Trial," *Journal of the American College of Nutrition* (2021), doi:10.1080/07315724.2020.1869625.

12. Klodian Dhana, Denis A. Evans, Kumar B. Rajan et al., "Healthy Lifestyle and the Risk of Alzheimer Dementia: Findings From 2 Longitudinal Studies." *Neurology* 95, no. 4 (July 2020): e374–e383, doi:10.1212/WNL.0000000000009816.

13. Seema Mihrshahi, Ding Ding, Joanne Gale et al., "Vegetarian Diet and All-Cause Mortality: Evidence From a Large Population-Based Australian Cohort—The 45 and Up Study." *Preventive Medicine* 97 (April 2017): 1–7, doi:10.1016/j.ypmed.2016.12.044.

14. George W. Rebok, Karlene Ball, Lin T. Guey et al., "Ten-Year Effects of the Advanced Cognitive Training for Independent and Vital Elderly Cognitive Training Trial on Cognition and Everyday Functioning in Older Adults," *Journal of the American Geriatrics Society* 62, no. 1 (2014): 16–24, doi:10.1111/jgs.12607.

15. Bruno Bonnechère, Christelle Langley, and Barbara Jacquelyn Sahakian, "The Use of Commercial Computerised Cognitive Games in Older Adults: A Meta-Analysis," *Scientific Reports* 10, article no. 15276 (2020), doi:10.1038/s41598-020-72281-3.

16. P. Pazos, Y. Leira, C. Domínguez et al., "Association Between Periodontal Disease and Dementia: A Literature Review," *Neurología* 33, issue 9 (November–December 2018): 602–613, doi:10.1016/j .nrleng.2016.07.007.

17. Marjo H. Eskelinen, Tiia Ngandu, Jaakko Tuomilehto et al., "Midlife Coffee and Tea Drinking and the Risk of Late-Life Dementia: A Population-Based CAIDE Study," *Journal of Alzheimer's Disease* 16, no. 1 (2009): 85–91, doi: 10.3233/JAD-2009-0920. See also: Oregon State University, Linus Pauling Institute, Micronutrient Information Center, "Coffee," https://lpi.oregon state.edu/mic/food-beverages/coffee#adverse-effects.

18. Wojciech Grodzicki and Katarzyna Dziendzikowska, "The Role of Selected Bioactive Compounds in the Prevention of Alzheimer's Disease," *Antioxidants* 9, no. 3 (2020): 229, doi:10.3390/ antiox9030229.

19. Michael F. Roizen and Michael C. Crupain, *What to Eat When: A Strategic Plan to Improve Your Health & Life Through Food* (Washington, D.C.: National Geographic, 2019).

20. Min Wei, Sebastian Brandorst, Mahshid Shelehchi et al., "Fasting-Mimicking Diet and Markers/ Risk Factors for Aging, Diabetes, Cancer, and Cardiovascular Disease," *Science Translational Medicine* 9, no. 377 (2017): eaai8700, doi:10.1126/scitranslmed.aai8700.

21. Rafael de Cabo and Mark P. Mattson, "Effects of Intermittent Fasting on Health, Aging, and Disease," *New England Journal of Medicine* 381, no. 26 (2019): 2541–2551, doi:10.1056/NEJMra1905136.

22. Timo E. Strandberg, Arto Strandberg, Kaisu Pitkälä et al., "Sauna Bathing, Health, and Quality of Life Among Octogenarian Men: The Helsinki Businessmen Study," *Aging Clinical and Experimental Research* 30, no. 9 (2018): 1053–1057, doi:10.1007/s40520-017-0855-z.

23. Maria D. Bernat-Adell, Eladio J. Collado-Boira, Pilar Moles-Julio et al., "Recovery of Inflammation, Cardiac, and Muscle Damage Biomarkers After Running a Marathon," *The Journal of Strength & Conditioning Research* 35, no. 3 (2021): 626–632, doi:10.1519/ JSC.0000000000003167.

Sources

24. Ming-Hsien Chiang, Hau-Hsin Wu, Chia-Jen Shih et al., "Association Between Influenza Vaccination and Reduced Risks of Major Adverse Cardiovascular Events in Elderly Patient," *American Heart Journal* 193 (November 2017): 1–7, doi:10.1016/j.ahj.2017.07.020.

25. Hamid Mohseni, Amit Kiran, Reza Khorshidi et al., "Influenza Vaccination and Risk of Hospitalization in Patients With Heart Failure: A Self-Controlled Case Series Study," *European Heart Journal* 38, no. 5 (February 2017): 326–333, doi:10.1093/eurheartj/ehw411.

26. Philip C. Calder, Anitra C. Carr, Adrian F. Gombart et al., "Optimal Nutritional Status for a Well-Functioning Immune System Is an Important Factor to Protect Against Viral Infections," *Nutrients* 12, no. 4 (2020): 1181, doi:10.3390/nu12041181.

27. Karine Spiegel, John F. Sheridan, and Eve Van Cauter, "Effect of Sleep Deprivation on Response to Immunization," *JAMA* 288, no. 12 (2002): 1471–1472.

28. Michael F. Roizen, *This Is Your Do-Over: The 7 Secrets to Losing Weight, Living Longer, and Getting a Second Chance at the Life You Want* (New York: Scribner, 2016).

29. S. Fu, C. L. Thompson, A. Ali et al., "Mechanical Loading Inhibits Cartilage Inflammatory Signalling Via an HDAC6 and IFT-Dependent Mechanism Regulating Primary Cilia Elongation," *Osteoarthritis and Cartilage* 27, no. 7 (July 1, 2019): 1064–1074, doi:10.1016/j.joca.2019.03.003.

30. Arch G. Mainous III, Rebecca J. Tanner, Kiarash P. Rahmanian et al., "Effect of Sedentary Lifestyle on Cardiovascular Disease Risk Among Healthy Adults With Body Mass Indexes 18.5 to 29.9 kg/m²," *The American Journal of Cardiology* 123, no. 5 (March 1, 2019): 764–768, doi:10.1016/j.amjcard.2018.11.043.

31. Francesca Saladini and Paolo Palatini, "Arterial Distensibility, Physical Activity, and the Metabolic Syndrome," *Current Hypertension Reports* 20, article no. 39 (2018), doi:10.1007/s11906-018-0837-3.

32. Brett R. Gordon, Cillian P. McDowell, Mats Hallgren et al., "Association of Efficacy of Resistance Exercise Training With Depressive Symptoms: Meta-Analysis and Meta-Regression Analysis of Randomized Clinical Trials," *JAMA Psychiatry* 75, no. 6 (2018): 566–576, doi:10.1001/jamapsychiatry.2018.0572.

33. Magdalena I. Tolea and James E. Galvin, "Sarcopenia and Impairment in Physical and Cognitive Functionality," *Clinical Interventions in Aging* 10 (2015): 663–671, doi:10.2147/CIA.S76275.

34. Kyle Mandsager, Serge Harb, Paul Cremer et al., "Association of Cardiorespiratory Fitness With Long-Term Mortality Among Adults Undergoing Exercise Treadmill Testing," *JAMA Network Open* 1, no. 6 (2018): e183605, doi:10.1001/jamanetworkopen.2018.3605.

35. Larry A. Tucker, J. Eric Strong, James D. LeCheminant et al., "Effect of Two Jumping Programs on Hip Bone Mineral Density in Premenopausal Women: A Randomized Controlled Trial," *American Journal of Health Promotion* 29, no. 3 (2015): 158–164, doi:10.4278/ajhp.130430-QUAN-200.

36. Alexander G. Robling, Felicia M. Hinant, David B. Burr et al., "Shorter, More Frequent Mechanical Loading Sessions Enhance Bone Mass," *Medicine & Science in Sports & Exercise* 34, no. 2 (2002): 196–202, doi:10.1097/00005768-200202000-00003.

37. Rubina Manuela Trimboli, Marina Codari, Marco Guazzi et al., "Screening Mammography

Beyond Breast Cancer: Breast Arterial Calcifications as a Sex-Specific Biomarker of Cardiovascular Risk," *European Journal of Radiology* 119 (2019): 108636.

38. Sofie Pardaens, Anne-Marie Willems, Els Clays et al., "The Impact of Drop-Out in Cardiac Rehabilitation on Outcome Among Coronary Artery Disease Patients," *European Journal of Preventive Cardiology* 24, no. 14 (2017): 1490–1497. doi:10.1177/2047487317724574.

39. Andrea Gurmankin Levy, Aaron M. Scherer, Brian J. Zikmund-Fisher et al., "Prevalence of and Factors Associated With Patient Nondisclosure of Medically Relevant Information to Clinicians," *JAMA Network Open* 1, no. 7 (2018): e185293, doi:10.1001/jamanetworkopen.2018.5293.

40. Nicholas J. Thomas, Anita L. Lynam, Anita V. Hill et al., "Type 1 Diabetes Defined by Severe Insulin Deficiency Occurs After 30 Years of Age and Is Commonly Treated as Type 2 Diabetes," *Diabetologia* 62 (2019): 1167–1172, doi: 10.1007/s00125-019-4863-8.

41. Michael F. Roizen and Mehmet C. Oz, *YOU: The Smart Patient. An Insider's Handbook for Getting the Best Treatment* (New York: Scribner, 2006).

42. Katherine Eban, *Bottle of Lies: The Inside Story of the Generic Drug Boom*, reprint edition (New York: Ecco Press / HarperCollins, 2020).

CHAPTER 14

1. David Brooks, "The Moral Bucket List," *New York Times*, April 11, 2015.

2. M. E. Camacho and C. A. Reyes-Ortiz, "Sexual Dysfunction in the Elderly: Age or Disease?" *International Journal of Impotence Research* 17 (2005): S52–S56, doi: 10.1038/sj.ijir.3901429.

3. Naveen R. Parva, Satish Tadepalli, Pratiksha Singh et al., "Prevalence of Vitamin D Deficiency and Associated Risk Factors in the US Population (2011–2012)," *Cureus* 10, no. 6 (2018): e2741, doi: 10.7759/cureus.2741.

4. William B. Grant, Fatme Al Anouti, and Meis Moukayed, "Targeted 25-Hydroxyvitamin D Concentration Measurements and Vitamin D_3 Supplementation Can Have Important Patient and Public Health Benefits," *European Journal of Clinical Nutrition* 74 (2020): 366–376, doi:10.1038/s41430-020-0564-0.

5. Amir S. Heravi and Erin D. Michos, "Vitamin D and Calcium Supplements: Helpful, Harmful, or Neutral for Cardiovascular Risk?" *Methodist Debakey Cardiovascular Journal* 15, no. 3 (July–September 2019): 207–213.

6. J. Michael Gaziano, Howard D. Sesso, William G. Christen et al., "Multivitamins in the Prevention of Cancer in Men: The Physicians' Health Study II Randomized Controlled Trial," *JAMA* 308, no. 18 (2012): 1871–1880, doi:10.1001/jama.2012.14641.

7. Kimberly Y. Z. Forrest and Wendy L. Stuhldreher, "Prevalence and Correlates of Vitamin D Deficiency in US Adults," *Nutrition Research* 31, no. 1 (2011): 48–54, doi:10.1016/j.nutres.2010.12.001.

8. Susanne Rautiainen, Pamela M. Rist, Robert J. Glynn et al., "Multivitamin Use and the Risk of Cardiovascular Disease in Men." *Journal of Nutrition* 146, no. 6 (June 2016): 1235–1240, doi:10.3945/jn.115.227884.

9. Mariann Fagernaes Hansen, Sarah Østrup Jensen, Ernst-Martin Füchtbauer et al., "High Folic Acid Diet Enhances Tumour Growth in PyMT-Induced Breast Cancer," *British Journal of Cancer* 116 (2017): 752–761, doi:10.1038/bjc.2017.11.

Sources

10. Jose L. Flores-Guerrero, Isidor Minović, Dion Groothof et al., "Association of Plasma Concentration of Vitamin B$_{12}$ With All-Cause Mortality in the General Population in the Netherlands." *JAMA Network Open* 3, no. 1 (2020): e1919274, doi:10.1001/jamanetwork open.2019.19274.

11. Edward Giovannucci, Yan Liu, Meir J. Stampfer et al., "A Prospective Study of Calcium Intake and Incident and Fatal Prostate Cancer," *Cancer Epidemiology, Biomarkers & Prevention* 15, no. 2 (2006): 203–210, doi:10.1158/1055-9965.EPI-05-0586.

12. Mohammad Al Qadire, Murad Alkhalaileh, and Hedaya Hina, "Risk Factors for Breast Cancer Among Jordanian Women: A Case-Control Study," *Iran Journal of Public Health* 47, no. 1 (January 2018): 49–56.

13. Jürgen Kern, Silke Kern, Kaj Blennow et al., "Calcium Supplementation and Risk of Dementia in Women With Cerebrovascular Disease," *Neurology* 87, no. 16 (October 2016): 1674–1680, doi:10.1212/WNL.0000000000003111.

14. Karin Yurko-Mauro, Deanna McCarthy, Dror Rom et al., "Beneficial Effects of Docosahexaenoic Acid on Cognition in Age-Related Cognitive Decline," *Alzheimer's & Dementia* 6, no. 6 (2010): 456–464, doi:10.1016/j.jalz.2010.01.013.

15. Ian Yat Hin Wong, Simon Chi Yan Koo, and Clement Wai Nangg Chan, "Prevention of Age-Related Macular Degeneration," *International Ophthalmology* 31 (2011): 73–82, doi:10.1007/s10792-010-9397-5.

16. Kelvin Tsoi, Jason M. W. Ho, Felix C. H. Chan et al., "Long-Term Use of Low-Dose Aspirin for Cancer Prevention: A 10-Year Population Cohort Study in Hong Kong," *International Journal of Cancer* 145, no. 1 (2019): 267–273, doi:10.1002/ijc.32083.

17. Michael F. Roizen and Mehmet C. Oz, *YOU: Staying Young: The Owner's Manual to Extending Your Warranty* (New York: Scribner, 2008).

18. Raymond John Playford and Michael James Weiser, "Bovine Colostrum: Its Constituents and Uses," *Nutrients* 13, no. 1 (2021): 265, doi:10.3390/nu13010265.

19. In-Bong Song, Hyejung Gu, Hye-Ju Han et al., "Omega-7 Inhibits Inflammation and Promotes Collagen Synthesis Through SIRT1 Activation," *Applied Biological Chemistry* 61 (2018): 433–439, doi:10.1007/s13765-018-0377-1.

20. Zeneng Wang, Nathalie Bergeron, Bruce S Levison et al., "Impact of Chronic Dietary Red Meat, White Meat, or Non-Meat Protein on Trimethylamine N-Oxide Metabolism and Renal Excretion in Healthy Men and Women," *European Heart Journal* 40, no. 7 (February 14, 2019): 583–594, doi:10.1093/eurheartj/ehy799.

21. W. H. Wilson Tang, Xinmin S. Li, Yuping Wu et al., "Plasma Trimethylamine N-oxide (TMAO) Levels Predict Future Risk of Coronary Artery Disease in Apparently Healthy Individuals in the EPIC-Norfolk Prospective Population Study," *American Heart Journal* (2021), doi:10.1016/j.ahj.2021.01.020.

22. Feilong Deng, Ying Li, and Jiangchao Zhao, "The Gut Microbiome of Healthy Long-Living People," *Aging* 11, no. 2 (January 15, 2019): 289–290, doi:10.18632/aging.101771.

23. Francisco M. Gutierrez-Mariscal, Elena M. Yubero-Serrano, Jose M. Villalba et al., "Coenzyme Q10: From Bench to Clinic in Aging Diseases, a Translational Review," *Critical Reviews in Food Science and Nutrition* 59, no. 14 (2019): 2240–2257, doi:10.1080/10408398.2018.1442316.

24. Alma Martelli, Lara Testai, Alessandro Colletti et al., "Coenzyme Q_{10}: Clinical Applications in Cardiovascular Diseases," *Antioxidants* 9, no. 4 (2020): 341, doi.org/10.3390/antiox9040341.

25. Mukesh K. Jain and Paul M. Ridker, "Anti-Inflammatory Effects of Statins: Clinical Evidence and Basic Mechanisms," *Nature Reviews Drug Discovery* 4 (2005): 977–987, doi:10.1038/nrd1901.

26. Emmanuel Maheu, Christian Cadet, Marc Marty et al., "Randomised, Controlled Trial of Avocado-Soybean Unsaponifiable (Piascledine) Effect on Structure Modification in Hip Osteoarthritis: The ERADIAS Study," *Annals of the Rheumatic Diseases* 73, no. 2 (February 2014): 376–384, doi:10.1136/annrheumdis-2012-202485.

27. Blaine A. Christiansen, Simrit Bhatti, Ramin Goudarzi et al., "Management of Osteoarthritis With Avocado/Soybean Unsaponifiables," *Cartilage* 6, no. 1 (2015): 30–44, doi:10.1177/1947603514554992.

28. Keisuke Hikosaka, Keisuke Yaku, Keisuke Okabe et al., "Implications of NAD Metabolism in Patho-physiology and Therapeutics for Neurodegenerative Diseases," *Nutritional Neuroscience* (2019): 1–13, doi:10.1080/1028415X.2019.1637504.

29. Ozlem Altay, Muhammad Arif, Xiangyu Li et al., "Combined Metabolic Activators Accelerates Recovery in Mild-to-Moderate COVID-19," *medRxiv* (2020), doi:10.1101/2020.10.02.20202614.

30. Mahsa Hatami, Mina Abdolahi, Neda Soveyd et al., "Molecular Mechanisms of Curcumin in Neuro-inflammatory Disorders: A Mini Review of Current Evidences," *Endocrine, Metabolic & Immune Disorders—Drug Targets* 19, no. 3 (2019): 247–258, doi:10.2174/1871530319666181129103056.

31. Javad Sharifi-Rad, Youssef El Rayess, Alain Abi Rizk et al., "Turmeric and Its Major Compound Curcumin on Health: Bioactive Effects and Safety Profiles for Food, Pharmaceutical, Biotechno-logical and Medicinal Applications," *Frontiers in Pharmacology* 11 (2020): 01021, doi:10.3389/fphar.2020.01021.

32. WebMD, "Turmeric," https://www.webmd.com/vitamins/ai/ingredientmono-662/turmeric (accessed February 24, 2021).

33. Kiran Chaudhari, Conner D. Reynolds, and Shao-Hua Yang, "Metformin and Cognition From the Perspectives of Sex, Age, and Disease," *GeroScience* 42 (2020): 97–116, doi:10.1007/s11357-019-00146-3.

34. Ameya S. Kulkarni, Siram Gubbi, and Nir Barzilai, "Benefits of Metformin in Attenuating the Hallmarks of Aging," *Cell Metabolism* 32, no. 1 (2020): 15–30, doi:10.1016/j.cmet.2020.04.001.

35. Adam R. Konopka, Jaime L. Laurin, Hayden M. Schoenberg et al., "Metformin Inhibits Mitochondrial Adaptations to Aerobic Exercise Training in Older Adults," *Aging Cell* 18, no. 1 (2019): e12880, doi:10.1111/acel.12880.

36. Ralph DeFronzo, G. Alexander Fleming, Kim Chen et al., "Metformin-Associated Lactic Acidosis: Current Perspectives on Causes and Risk," *Metabolism* 65, no. 2 (2016): 20–29, doi:10.1016/j.metabol.2015.10.014.

37. Duncan Chambers, Anna J. Cantrell, Maxine Johnson et al., "Digital and Online Symptom Checkers and Health Assessment/Triage Services for Urgent Health Problems: Systematic Review," *BMJ Open* 9, no. 8 (2019): e027743, doi:10.1136/bmjopen-2018-027743.

38. Michael F. Roizen and Mehmet C. Oz, *YOU: Being Beautiful. The Owner's Manual to Inner and Outer Beauty* (New York: Free Press, 2008).

Sources

39. U.S. Food and Drug Administration, "FDA Advances New Proposed Regulation to Make Sure That Sunscreens Are Safe and Effective," February 21, 2019, https://www.fda.gov/news-events/press -announcements/fda-advances-new-proposed-regulation-make-sure-sunscreens-are-safe-and -effective.

40. Bagus Komang Satriyasa, "Botulinum Toxin (Botox) A for Reducing the Appearance of Facial Wrinkles: A Literature Review of Clinical Use and Pharmacological Aspect," *Clinical, Cosmetic and Investigational Dermatology* 12 (April 10, 2019): 223–228, doi:10.2147/CCID.S202919.

41. Larissa Rocha Bertelli Cabral, Lucas Novaes Teixeira, Rodrigo Pinto Gimenez et al., "Effect of Hyaluronic Acid and Poly-L-Lactic Acid Dermal Fillers on Collagen Synthesis: An In Vitro and In Vivo Study," *Clinical Cosmetic and Investigational Dermatology* 13 (September 29, 2020): 701–710, doi:10.2147/CCID.S266015.

42. Lloyd F. Rose and Rodney K. Chan, "The Burn Wound Microenvironment," *Advances in Wound Care* 5, no. 3 (2016): 106–118, doi:10.1089/wound.2014.0536.

43. Benjamin C. Marcus and David Hyman, "Evidence-Based Medicine in Laser Medicine for Facial Plastic Surgery," *Facial Plastic Surgery Clinics of North America* 23, no. 3 (2015): 297–302, doi:10.1016/ j.fsc.2015.04.003.

44. Fabio Santanelli di Pompeo, Michail Sorotos, Mark W. Clemens et al., "Breast Implant–Associated Anaplastic Large Cell Lymphoma (BIA-ALCL): Review of Epidemiology and Prevalence Assessment in Europe," *Aesthetic Surgery Journal* (2020): sjaa285, doi:10.1093/asj/sjaa285.

45. Vasileios Theocharidis, Ioannis Katsaros, Emmanouil Sgouromallis et al., "Current Evidence on the Role of Smoking in Plastic Surgery Elective Procedures: A Systematic Review and Meta-Analysis," *Journal of Plastic, Reconstructive & Aesthetic Surgery* 71, no. 5 (2018): 624–636, doi:10.1016/j.bjps.2018.01.011.

46. Robert Singer, "Commentary On: Improvement in Brazilian Butt Lift (BBL) Safety With the Current Recommendations From ASERF, ASAPS, and ISAPS," *Aesthetic Surgery Journal* 40, no. 8 (2020): 871–873, doi:10.1093/asj/sjaa090.

AFTERWORD

1. Prateek Lohia, Shweta Kapur, Sindhuri Benjaram et al., "Metabolic Syndrome and Clinical Outcomes in Patients Infected With COVID-19: Does Age, Sex, and Race of the Patient With Metabolic Syndrome Matter?" *Journal of Diabetes* (2021), doi:10.1111/1753-0407.13157.

ABOUT THE AUTHORS

This book's three authors share the same stance when it comes to the Great Age Reboot: Not only are major medical advances here, but many more life-extenders and age-reducers are on their way. In fact, during the course of writing this book, we identified no fewer than 18 significant medical/scientific advances that emerged in just 14 fields of aging research—and these (plus more) are fluid, as they evolve and advance every day.

Longevity should not be something to fear but something to embrace, enjoy, and prosper in. We have chosen the latter, and that's our major guiding principle.

Peter Linneman: Peter is 71 and quite healthy. His father was dead at age 49 of a heart attack and smoked two packs a day his entire life. His mother, at age 70, was obese and in bad condition. She died at 95 but was a physical wreck for at least 25 years and a mental wreck for eight years. A retired economics professor, Peter continues to advise, serve on boards, lecture, write, invest, exercise vigorously daily, and travel. He maintains a fairly healthy diet, but it is a constant struggle. His RealAge (a marker of a biological age compared with a calendar age, which we explain on page 17) is 58, inflated by successfully replaced arthritic hips.

Albert Ratner: Albert was born in 1927. He is now in his 11th decade. In a period of two years between his 10th and 12th birthdays, his grandmother, grandfather, and uncle all passed away. By the time he was 13 years old, he was convinced he would never live more than a year longer. He is now 94 years old and finds it hard to believe. When he was born, his life expectancy was 57 years. He has now lived 36-plus years longer than that, an increase of over 63 percent.

He has 16 or 17 stents (he doesn't know which), works every day, and has paid into Social Security since he was a young child. He has seen enormous changes in longevity (it gets longer), diet (it gets worse—no salt!), and exercise (about the same) and has come to realize that everyone has a great role in their own health and the health of our country.

Albert is still able to do the things he loves and that are important to him. "My reason for writing this book is to help people understand that they too can share the greatest gift that we can wish for and that is the gift of more happy, healthy, and productive years," he says. "Over these decades through medicines, medical devices, and the skill of doctors, we have been given the opportunity to participate in the gift that keeps on giving—longevity. All the other disruptors have changed part of your life, but longevity changes everything. So longevity is going to be the greatest disruptor."

Michael F. Roizen: Dr. Mike (board certified in both anesthesia and internal medicine after graduation from the University of California at San Francisco because he wanted to run an intensive care unit) has spent his medical career helping people understand that life choices have the most profound effect on your health and longevity. As the developer of RealAge, he looked at and examined thousands of studies (over 52,000 by actual count as of 1998, and probably a multiple of that number in addition since then) to show the effect that life choices have on the age your body feels, looks, and acts, as opposed to calendar age. As the chief wellness officer of the Cleveland Clinic, Dr. Mike has also seen firsthand the economic and medical impact of getting a group of people to make significant lifestyle changes. He is 76 years old, with a RealAge of 56. "That's where we must team up together: Let medicine do what it does best—treat illness, and you take care of yourself, and, especially your brain. And you can do both—you have that power as your own genetic engineer. That's the key to making yourself able to fight off challenges and stay vibrant and younger for much longer."

INDEX

Index